RESISTANCE BAND WORKOUT FOR SENIORS

ACHIEVE YOUR GOALS FOR PERFECT HEALTH WITH RESISTANCE BAND TRAINING

Dwight Kenneth

© Copyright 2024 Dwight Kenneth

Resistance Band Workout for Seniors

Copyrights Notice

Limited Liability

Please note that the content of this book is based on personal experience and various information sources.

Although the author has made every effort to present accurate, up-to-date, reliable, and complete information in this book, they make no representations or warranties concerning the accuracy or completeness of the content of this book and specifically disclaim any implied warranties of merchantability or fitness for a particular purpose.

Your particular circumstances may not be suited to the example illustrated in this book; in fact, they likely will not be. You should use the information in this book at your own risk.

All trademarks, service marks, product names, and the characteristics of any names mentioned in this book are considered the property of their respective owners and are used only for reference. No endorsement is implied when we use one of these terms.

This book is only for personal use. Please note the information contained within this document is for educational and entertainment purposes only and no warranties of any kind are declared or implied. Readers acknowledge that the author is not engaging in the rendering of legal, financial, or professional advice.

Please consult a licensed professional before attempting any techniques outlined in this book. Nothing in this book is intended to replace common sense legal accounting, or professional advice and is meant only to inform. By reading this document, the reader agrees that under no circumstances is the author responsible for any losses, direct or indirect, which are incurred as a result of the use of the information contained within this document, including, but not limited to, errors, omissions, or inaccuracies.

Table of Contents

Introduction 10

Chapter 1: Understanding the Benefits of Resistance Band
Training for Seniors 12

Chapter 2: Getting Started 17

Chapter 3: Foundations of Resistance Band Exercises............ 23

Chapter 4: Basic Resistance Band Exercises for Seniors 34

Chapter 5: Progressive Workouts.. 56

Chapter 6: Targeted Workouts for Common Senior Health
Concerns 64

Chapter 7: Incorporating Cardiovascular Exercise with
Resistance Bands... 74

Chapter 8: Partner and Group Exercises................................. 80

Chapter 9: Setting Realistic Goals 91

Chapter 10: Conclusion.. 113

Extra Content.. 128

Introduction

Welcome to "Resistance Band Workout, for Seniors " a guide created to empower and support individuals in their years as they strive for health and vitality. Aging is a part of life. It doesn't mean sacrificing strength, flexibility, or overall well-being. Instead, it presents an opportunity to discover effective ways to stay active improve mobility and maintain independence.

This book acknowledges that not all exercise routines are suitable for every stage of life. With this in mind, we delve into the world of resistance band training—an accessible approach tailored specifically to meet the needs of individuals.

In the chapters, we will guide you through a series of exercises designed to boost strength enhance flexibility, and promote health—all using resistance bands. These simple powerful tools offer an effective way for seniors to engage in a full-body workout without relying on heavy weights or complicated machinery.

Before we see the exercises, we'll explore the benefits that resistance band training can bring to senior's lives. You need to understand how this approach can have an impact, on your well-being. Ensuring safety is of importance so we will offer precautions and guidelines to make sure your workouts are enjoyable and free, from injuries. Regardless of whether you may be a fitness enthusiast or a person just starting their journey towards a healthier lifestyle, this book is designed to suit your current level. Experience the delight of movement regain confidence in your abilities and embark on a fitness journey that's not only effective but also sustainable in the long term. Get ready to embrace a chapter filled with vitality, strength, and overall well-being. Together let's embark on this journey—one resistance band at a time.

Chapter 1: Understanding the Benefits of Resistance Band Training for Seniors

Resistance band training provides benefits that are specifically suited to meet the needs and capabilities of adults. As we age it becomes increasingly important to maintain muscle mass and strength for our health and independence. Resistance bands offer a gentle way to engage in strength-building exercises without putting excessive strain on joints or risking injury. They can be adjusted according to fitness levels allowing older adults to progress at their pace and personalize their workouts based on individual requirements. Resistance band exercises are very important both for strength and because they promote flexibility, improve mobility, and reduce the risk of falls and various injuries which are a very common concern among older adults. Moreover, resistance band workouts have gained a reputation, for their impact on balance and stability which ultimately boosts confidence in activities. In this section, we will explore the benefits of incorporating resistance bands into your fitness routine. These advantages contribute to well-being and help create an active and fulfilling lifestyle as you gracefully navigate through the golden years.

Additionally, resistance bands offer a cost-effective alternative to gym equipment. Seniors can easily integrate these portable bands into their home exercise regimen removing any obstacles typically associated with going to the gym. The versatility of resistance bands allows for a range of exercises that target muscle groups resulting in a comprehensive full-body workout. This adaptability in exercise selection caters to individuals, with fitness levels and health conditions making it an inclusive and flexible fitness solution.

One remarkable aspect of resistance band training is its ability to provide resistance throughout the range of motion during an exercise. This continuous tension effectively engages muscles leading to strength gains and improved endurance. As we delve into resistance band exercises in sections you will discover how this dynamic training approach can enhance your functional capacity making everyday activities more manageable and enjoyable.

Moreover, the beauty of resistance band exercises lies in their impact, on joints making them an excellent choice for seniors dealing with arthritis or related issues. Whether you are a beginner who wants to start doing fitness or someone experienced seeking alternative resistance bands provide a safe and accessible solution.

Essentially this section aims to highlight the benefits of including resistance band training in your fitness routine. By understanding these advantages you'll feel more confident and enthusiastic about adopting this form of exercise ultimately fostering a more active lifestyle as you embrace the changes that come with aging.

Safety Considerations and Precautions

When embarking on any fitness journey as a senior prioritizing safety is crucial for an injury-free experience. While resistance band training is generally safe and accessible there are considerations to keep in mind to maximize its benefits. It's highly recommended to consult with a healthcare before starting any exercise program especially if you have pre-existing health conditions or concerns.

To avoid strain or injury while using resistance bands it's important to maintain form and technique. Each exercise outlined in this guide includes instructions, on maintaining posture, movement patterns, and breathing techniques.

Please read these instructions carefully before you begin, making sure you fully understand their meaning. Begin with a resistance level that's not too challenging so you can focus on getting the form. Once you've mastered that you can gradually increase the resistance.

It's important to choose the level of resistance based on your fitness level. If the band offers resistance it can strain your muscles. On the other hand, if it offers little resistance you may not get the desired workout intensity. Thanks to this book you will be able to understand how to select the right resistance for each exercise that is right for you so that you can personalize and adapt your training routine according to your goals. Just like with any exercise routine listen to your body. If you feel any pain (from discomfort, during a challenging workout) stop the exercise and check your form or switch to a band with lower resistance. Consistency is important. It's also crucial to give your body time to adapt and recover.

In the following sections, we will explore exercises. Structured workouts are designed for different levels of intensity. Safety and well-being are always our priorities. By keeping these factors in mind you'll be well prepared for a resistance band training journey that focuses on preventing injuries and meets your needs as a senior.

In addition, if you are a senior, with health concerns or chronic conditions it's advisable to consult with a therapist or certified fitness professional for personalized guidance and modifications tailored to your individual needs. These experts can give you insights on how to adapt resistance band exercises based on your mobility limitations, joint issues, or other health considerations ensuring that your workout routine is safe and customized.

Creating an exercise environment is also important. Choose an area with lighting free from any obstacles. Make sure you have a sturdy chair or support surface nearby if necessary. This will enhance stability during exercises. Minimize the risk of falls.

Including warm-up and cool-down routines in your exercise program is crucial when it comes to resistance band training. This guide will provide recommendations for up exercises to prepare your muscles and joints before the workout session as well as cooldown exercises that promote flexibility and aid in muscle recovery.

Lastly, remember to stay hydrated and listen to your body's signals. Dehydration can impact your energy levels. Increase the chance of experiencing cramps. Therefore it's vital to drink water during and, after your workout routine. If you start feeling lightheaded have difficulty breathing or experience any symptoms while exercising it's important to stop and seek medical attention if needed.

By incorporating these safety measures and precautions into your resistance band workouts you do not prioritize your well-being. Also, create an environment that promotes long-term success. As we go through this guide you'll discover how focusing on safety enhances the enjoyment and effectiveness of your resistance band training.

Chapter 2: Getting Started

In the "Getting Started" section we lay the groundwork, for your resistance band training journey. Here we provide steps to ensure a safe beginning to your fitness adventure. From choosing the resistance bands to setting up a workout area we cover the initial aspects that pave the way for a successful and gratifying experience. Whether you're new to exercise or an experienced fitness enthusiast exploring an approach this section equips you with the tools and knowledge to kickstart your resistance band training for seniors. Let's embark on this journey together as we take those steps toward improved strength, flexibility, and overall well-being.

Choosing the Right Resistance Bands

Choosing the resistance bands is an aspect, of crafting a personalized and efficient workout routine. In this guide, we aim to simplify the range of resistance bands available providing insights to assist you in making informed decisions based on your fitness level and personal needs. From bands to looped bands with levels of resistance, we will explore the unique features of each type and offer recommendations for seniors who want to safely build strength and improve flexibility.

The right choice of resistance band does not enhance the effectiveness of your exercises. Also contributes to a positive and enjoyable fitness journey. Let's dive into the world of resistance bands empowering you to select the tool for your path towards a healthier and more active lifestyle.

In the section titled "Choosing the Right Resistance Bands " our focus is on guiding seniors through the process of selecting the resistance bands for their workouts. This paragraph emphasizes the significance of making informed decisions based on fitness levels and specific needs. Here's a breakdown:

Demystifying Variety: there are types of resistance bands including flat bands and looped bands with different levels of resistance.

Informed Choices: our goal is to help readers make choices by understanding the characteristics associated with each type of resistance band and how they align with seniors' specific requirements. We aim to empower individuals, in choosing bands that suit their fitness goals and abilities.

Creating an Optimal Workout Environment: When it comes to resistance band training, for seniors "Setting Up a Comfortable Workout Space" emphasizes the significance of establishing an environment that prioritizes safety, comfort, and a positive overall experience. It highlights the importance of seniors feeling secure and at ease while engaging in resistance band exercises. By ensuring a workout space seniors can enhance their fitness journey. Make the most out of their resistance band workouts. Here's a breakdown of the content;

Prioritizing Safety: This phrase emphasizes the importance of considering safety when incorporating resistance band exercises into a fitness routine. It involves selecting a workout space that minimizes hazards and reduces the risk of accidents or injuries.

Sufficient Lighting: Ensuring lighting, in the exercise area is crucial for seniors. Good visibility helps them stay aware of their surroundings maintain form during exercises and reduce the risk of tripping or stumbling.

Clear Space: The workout area should be free from any clutter, obstacles, or objects that could potentially cause harm during exercise. This allows seniors to move freely without worrying about tripping over things creating an environment for their workouts.

Stable Support Surface: Seniors may find it beneficial to have a chair or support surface nearby for exercises that involve sitting or require added stability. This provides an option for support if needed during movements.

Comfortable Environment: In addition to safety it's important to create an inviting atmosphere for workouts. Factors such as room temperature, ventilation, and ensuring that the exercise area promotes an enjoyable and positive experience are essential.

Accessibility: The setup should be easily accessible, to seniors considering any mobility limitations they may have.

To set up a comfortable workout space there are steps you can take. First, make sure that resistance bands are easily accessible. Next, consider the mobility aids that may be needed and ensure that the exercise area can accommodate them. Lastly make any adjustments, to the setup based on needs.

In addition to these considerations, it's important to incorporate preferences into the workout space. Encourage seniors to personalize their environment with things that they enjoy. This could include playing their music having a water bottle for hydration or adding elements that create a pleasant atmosphere.

In summary, creating a comfortable workout space for seniors involves prioritizing safety minimizing hazards, and promoting overall comfort during resistance band training. It's about making sure that the exercise area is conducive to an experience while also considering needs and preferences.

Proper Warm-up and Cool-down Techniques

The significance of " Warm up and Cool down Techniques", in the context of "Resistance Band Training for Seniors" cannot be overstated. It emphasizes the importance of preparing the body before a workout and facilitating recovery afterward. Here's a breakdown:

Preventing Injury: This concept acknowledges that a proper warm-up is vital to ready the body for the exercise regimen. For seniors, who may require time to adjust it's crucial to have a warm-up routine that increases blood flow to the muscles enhances joint flexibility, and minimizes injury risks during resistance band exercises.

Dynamic Stretching: Warm-ups often incorporate dynamic stretching exercises that gently engage muscle groups. These movements gradually elevate senior's heart rates warm up their muscles and improve flexibility creating a condition for workouts.

Specificity to Resistance Bands: The guide likely offers up techniques specifically designed for resistance band training. This could involve incorporating resistance band exercises or mimicking movements to those in the main workout session effectively preparing the muscles, for targeted exercises.

Mind-Body Connection: Warm-ups play a role in helping seniors establish a connection between their mind and body. During this time they can focus on maintaining form regulating their breathing and mentally preparing themselves for the workout. This mindfulness greatly contributes to ensuring a more effective exercise session.

Cool-down for Recovery: It's important to emphasize the significance of incorporating a cool-down routine for seniors to aid in their recovery process. After completing the workout seniors are guided through exercises that gradually lower their heart rate prevent blood from pooling in their extremities and promote relaxation.

Static Stretching: Cooldowns often include stretching exercises which are beneficial for improving flexibility and reducing muscle stiffness. These stretches involve holding positions for a period helping to maintain joint mobility and muscle elasticity.

Promoting Flexibility and Range of Motion: The ultimate goal is to enhance flexibility and ensure seniors maintain a range of motion in their joints. These factors are particularly crucial, for preventing injuries improving mobility, and supporting health among seniors.

In summary, "Proper Warm-up and Cool-down Techniques" in the context of resistance band training for seniors involves providing guidance on specific warm-up exercises tailored to resistance band workouts, emphasizing the importance of preventing injury, and incorporating effective cool-down techniques for recovery and flexibility maintenance.

Chapter 3: Foundations of Resistance Band Exercises

In the section titled "Foundations of Resistance Band Exercise," we explore the principles that are essential for safe and effective resistance band training for seniors. This section is crucial as it provides insights into grip and hand positions highlights the significance of maintaining body alignment and posture and emphasizes controlled breathing to maximize the benefits of resistance band exercises. By understanding these elements you will establish a foundation for a satisfying fitness journey that is free from injuries. Let's now delve into the components that form the basis of resistance band training empowering you with confidence and expertise as you embark on your fitness journey.

Grip and Hand Positions

In resistance band training specifically designed for seniors, we cannot underestimate the importance of grip and hand positions. These foundational elements serve as the basis, for exercise routines while contributing to both muscle engagement and overall success and enjoyment during workouts.

In this guide, we will delve into the intricacies of grip and hand positions breaking down the elements that seniors should grasp and master to optimize their resistance band training experience.

Understanding the Basics. Before getting into the specifics it's crucial to understand the principles that govern grip and hand positions when working with resistance bands. Unlike weights or machines, resistance bands offer a form of resistance that demands a deliberate and controlled approach. The elasticity of the bands adds an aspect, to your workout routine requiring you to be mindful of how you place your hands and the strength you apply to activate your muscles effectively while keeping your joints safe.

Types of Resistance Bands. The type of resistance band you use can influence the grip and hand positions. Different bands like bands looped bands or figure eight bands have characteristics that require different approaches. For example, with bands, it's often recommended to hold them with a hand grip while looped bands might require wrapping them around your hands or wrists. Understanding these variations is essential as it helps you choose the grip, for each type of resistance band you're using—enhancing both effectiveness and comfort during exercises.

Proper Grip Techniques. Establishing a proper grip forms the foundation for a resistance band workout. Seniors should focus on achieving a comfortable grip avoiding any tension, in their hands or fingers. When using bands it's common to hold the band with a hand and spread the fingers comfortably apart. Loop bands may require wrapping them around the hands or wrists while maintaining controlled tension. It's essential to emphasize the importance of maintaining this grip throughout the exercise for muscle engagement and overall safety.

Hand Positions and Alignment. Hand positions play a role in targeting muscle groups and ensuring proper body alignment during resistance band exercises. To minimize stress on joints and optimize muscle recruitment it is generally recommended to maintain a wrist position. Whether performing bicep curls, shoulder presses, or leg exercises seniors should be mindful of keeping their wrists in a position to prevent strain and potential discomfort.

Adaptions for Joint Health. When it comes to health seniors who may be more prone to sensitivities can benefit from certain adaptations in grip and hand positions during resistance band exercises. For individuals with arthritis or joint discomfort using handles or grips designed for support can enhance comfort. Reduce strain. Exploring variations that accommodate needs ensures that resistance band training remains accessible and enjoyable for seniors, at fitness levels and health conditions.

Integrating Hand and Finger Exercises. In addition, to the resistance band workouts seniors can include hand and finger exercises in their routine to improve grip strength and dexterity. These exercises, like squeezing fingers or stretching hands not enhance the effectiveness of resistance band training. Also, promotes overall hand health. Strengthening the hands can make daily activities easier. Add an aspect to a senior's fitness regimen.

Breathing Synchronization. One aspect often overlooked in resistance band training is synchronizing breathing with grip and hand movements. Proper breathing improves stability and supports muscle engagement. Helps maintain control during exercises. Seniors are encouraged to develop a breathing pattern that complements their movements creating a mind-body connection that enhances the effectiveness of resistance band workouts.

Progression and Variations. As seniors become more familiar with grip and hand positions, in resistance band exercises it's important to introduce progression and variations. Gradually increasing resistance levels trying out hand positions and exploring exercises ensures a dynamic and challenging workout routine. This progressive approach does not prevent stagnation. Also keeps seniors motivated on their fitness journey.

Troubleshooting and Common Errors. Seniors need to understand the mistakes associated with grip and hand positions to make the most of resistance band training while reducing the risk of injury. By addressing issues, like gripping incorrect wrist alignment or neglecting hand and finger health seniors can identify problems in their technique and make necessary adjustments for a safe and effective workout.

Conclusion of the Content " Grip and Hand Positions". In conclusion, the information on grip and hand positions in resistance band training for seniors goes beyond details. It forms the foundation of a fitness journey that empowers them. By mastering these elements seniors can unlock the potential of resistance band exercises promoting strength, flexibility, and overall well-being. This guide acts as a roadmap equipping seniors with knowledge and tools to navigate grip and hand positions with confidence as they pursue a more active lifestyle.

Body Alignment and Posture

When it comes to fitness having body alignment and posture is crucial for maximizing the benefits of resistance band training. Not do these aspects help prevent injuries. Also ensure that muscles are engaged efficiently during workouts, for optimal results. In this guide, we will explore the intricacies of body alignment and posture providing insights, to seniors on how to optimize their resistance band training experience and maintain a healthy and active lifestyle.

Understanding the Importance. Body alignment and posture are foundations for any exercise routine for seniors who engage in resistance band training. The way you position your body during exercises directly affects muscle engagement, joint stability, and overall safety. Seniors have considerations like sensitivities or balance concerns so paying close attention to alignment is essential for a successful and injury-free workout.

Foundations of Proper Alignment. Proper body alignment starts with establishing a foundation typically through a stable and well-aligned stance. When performing standing exercises it's recommended that seniors evenly distribute their weight between both feet to create a base. The alignment of the head, shoulders, and hips plays a role in promoting the curvature of the spine while minimizing strain and optimizing muscle recruitment.

Neutral Spine for Joint Health. A neutral spine is crucial for maintaining body alignment among seniors who may be more prone to spinal issues. Keeping a spine involves preserving the curves of your back, without excessive arching or rounding. Not only does proper alignment support health but it also helps in effectively transmitting force during resistance band exercises.

Adaptations for Seated Exercises. Acknowledging that not all older adults may feel comfortable doing standing exercises the guide offers adjustments to maintain alignment when performing seated exercises. Whether sitting in a chair or on the floor seniors are instructed on how to position their spine, pelvis, and limbs to ensure muscle engagement while minimizing the risk of strain.

Joint-Friendly Positions. When it comes to fitness joint health is often a consideration. Body alignment plays a role in creating positions that are gentle on joints during resistance band exercises. For instance, emphasizing alignment in the knees hips and ankles helps reduce stress on weight-bearing joints. This makes resistance band training accessible and beneficial for individuals with arthritis or joint concerns.

Mind-Body Connection. The guide emphasizes the importance of cultivating a mind-body connection, throughout resistance band exercises. Seniors are encouraged to be mindful of their body alignment feel their muscles engaging and pay attention to how different movements affect their posture. This heightened awareness does not enhance the effectiveness of the workout. Also improves overall body awareness. It contributes to balance and coordination.

Breathing Techniques and Posture. One aspect covered in the guide is the integration of breathing techniques, with maintaining good body alignment. Seniors are taught how synchronized breathing can improve their posture provide stability and give them a sense of control while doing resistance band exercises. This mindful approach to breathing works hand in hand with the movements creating a connection between the musculoskeletal systems.

Specifics for Different Exercises. The content provides information on body alignment and posture for various resistance band exercises. Whether seniors are doing upper body exercises like bicep curls or lower body exercises like leg presses they receive instructions on how to position their bodies for effectiveness. This attention to detail ensures that proper alignment is seamlessly incorporated into every aspect of their resistance band workout routine.

Progression and Adaptability. Recognizing that seniors have fitness levels and capabilities the guide introduces the concepts of progression and adaptability when it comes to maintaining body alignment. Seniors are guided on how to challenge themselves by incorporating complex movements while also being able to make adjustments based on their individual needs and limitations. This personalized approach ensures that maintaining body alignment remains a focus, throughout their fitness journey.

Troubleshooting Common Postural Mistakes. Acknowledging that mastering body alignment takes time the guide addresses common mistakes people may make with their posture and provides troubleshooting tips to overcome them. Seniors can identify and address issues like slouching or arching their back during resistance band exercises ensuring that they perform the movements accurately and safely.

Conclusion of the Content "Body Alignment and Posture". In conclusion, understanding and applying the principles of body alignment and posture is crucial, for seniors who are starting resistance band training. By incorporating these principles seniors can go beyond simply doing exercises and adopt an approach that improves muscle engagement, joint health, and overall well-being. This comprehensive guide provides seniors with the knowledge to navigate the nuances of body alignment enabling them to have a secure and effective experience, with resistance band training as they strive for a more active lifestyle.

Breathing Techniques, in "Resistance Band Workout for Seniors": A Comprehensive Guide

When it comes to resistance band training for seniors one aspect that often gets overlooked is the importance of breathing techniques. These techniques play a role in optimizing the effectiveness, safety, and overall enjoyment of workouts. In this guide, we'll explore the nuances of breathing techniques and how seniors can use breathing to enhance muscle engagement improve stability, and develop a mindful connection with their bodies.

The Breath-Movement Connection. Breathing goes beyond being a bodily function – it's a fundamental part of movement, especially in resistance band training. Understanding how breath and movement are interconnected is essential for seniors as they participate in exercises that target muscle groups. This guide sheds light on how synchronized breathing creates harmony between the musculoskeletal systems resulting in more controlled workout experiences.

Foundations of Proper Breathing. Proper breathing starts with understanding breathing, as its foundation. Seniors are encouraged to take breaths allowing their diaphragm to descend while their lungs fill with air. This technique does not maximize oxygen intake. Also engages the diaphragm and core muscles providing stability and support during resistance band exercises. Highlighting the significance of breathing through the nose especially when exerting oneself further optimizes the intake of oxygen. Helps regulate effort.

Inhalation and Exhalation Phases. The guide explains the phases of inhaling and exhaling in relation, to resistance band movements. For example, during the phase (when muscles shorten) of an exercise like lifting a resistance band seniors are advised to take deep breaths. On the other hand during the phase (when muscles lengthen) such as lowering the band a controlled exhale is recommended. This phased approach ensures that the respiratory system adequately supports each movement's demands, promoting efficiency while minimizing breath-holding risks that can increase tension and reduce stability.

Mindful Breath Control. Breath control goes beyond inhaling and exhaling; it encompasses being consciously aware of the rhythm and depth of one's breath. Seniors are encouraged to cultivate an awareness of their breathing paying attention to its quality and pace. This mindfulness strengthens the connection between mind and body allowing seniors to synchronize their breath with movement. It fosters a sense of control and stability during resistance band exercises.

Adaptations for Different Exercises. The guide offers adaptations, for incorporating breathing techniques into various resistance band exercises. Whether seniors are performing upper body exercises such, as bicep curls or lower body exercises like leg presses they receive guidance on how to coordinate their breathing with each movement. This adaptability ensures that breathing techniques seamlessly integrate into the various exercises seniors may engage in promoting a mindful approach throughout their workout routine.

Breath Awareness for Core Engagement. The engagement of core muscles is closely connected to proper breathing techniques. The guide emphasizes how intentional breathing can activate core muscles providing stability to the spine and enhancing posture. Seniors are encouraged to develop an awareness of how their breath impacts their core understanding that breath and core engagement work to support a strong and balanced body during resistance band training.

Enhancing Relaxation and Reducing Tension. Proper breathing techniques extend beyond the aspects of exercise; they also contribute to mental well-being by promoting relaxation and reducing tension. Seniors are urged to adopt rhythmic and calming breath patterns during their workouts creating an environment that not only optimizes performance but also fosters a positive and enjoyable exercise experience.

Breathing for Stress Reduction. Resistance band training can be an approach, for both mental well-being, which is why the guide introduces breathing techniques specifically designed for stress reduction. Seniors receive guidance in performing relaxation exercises that involve breaths. These exercises aim to reduce stress and foster a sense of calmness. This aspect acknowledges the connection, between fitness and mental well being recognizing how resistance band training can contribute to wellness.

Progression in Breath Awareness. Similar to how workout routines incorporate increasing levels of resistance the guide introduces a progression in breath awareness. Seniors are encouraged to begin with breath control techniques and gradually advance to complex breathing methods as they become more comfortable with the exercises. This approach aligns with the nature of resistance band training allowing seniors to adapt their breath control according to their evolving fitness levels.

Troubleshooting Common Breathing Mistakes. Recognizing that mastering breathing techniques takes time and practice the guide addresses mistakes. Provides troubleshooting tips. Seniors are empowered to identify and correct issues like breathing, breath holding, or irregular breathing patterns. This ensures that their resistance band exercises are not only effective but also performed with breath control.

Integration with Relaxation Techniques. The guide explores combining breathing techniques with relaxation exercises emphasizing the significance of workout recovery. Seniors are guided through deep breathing sequences and relaxation routines fostering an approach, to winding down after a resistance band workout. This integration helps seniors relax recover their muscles and improve their well-being.

Conclusion of the Content "Breathing Techniques, in "Resistance Band Workout for Seniors": A Comprehensive Guide". In conclusion, the information, about using breathing techniques in resistance band training for seniors highlights the impact of breathing. By understanding the basics practicing breath control and incorporating breathing into their workouts seniors can enhance their exercise experience. This comprehensive guide not only emphasizes the advantages of proper breathing but also recognizes its role in mental well promoting a holistic approach to senior fitness through resistance band training.

Chapter 4: Basic Resistance Band Exercises for Seniors

In the section on " Basic Resistance Band Exercises for Seniors," we explore movements that serve as the foundation of a well-rounded resistance band workout. Designed specifically with seniors in mind these exercises prioritize safety, effectiveness, and adaptability. From seated exercises to standing routines that enhance stability each movement is carefully crafted to enhance strength, flexibility, and overall mobility. Whether you're new to resistance band training or looking for a refresher course this section provides a starting point while empowering seniors to embrace the benefits of resistance band exercises with confidence and enthusiasm. Let's embark, on this accessible and invigorating fitness journey together.

Upper Body Exercises

The section, on "Upper Body Exercises" in the book "Resistance Band Training for Seniors" is a guide that aims to help older individuals perform safe resistance band workouts specifically targeting their upper body. This section takes into account the needs and considerations of seniors providing them with a roadmap to build strength improve flexibility and enhance mobility in their upper body.

Understanding the Importance of Upper Body Strength

Recognizing the importance of having body muscles this guide emphasizes how vital they are for seniors to maintain functional independence. Everyday activities like reaching for objects or carrying groceries heavily rely on the strength and flexibility of these muscles. By focusing on developing body strength seniors can better support themselves in their tasks and enjoy an improved overall quality of life.

Adaptability and Accessibility

To cater to seniors' diverse fitness levels and abilities the exercises chosen for this section have been carefully selected for their adaptability. Each exercise is designed to be adjusted according to fitness levels allowing seniors to progress at their pace while ensuring that the workouts remain accessible and safe. The goal is inclusivity, encouraging individuals with fitness backgrounds to participate in exercises tailored to meet their unique needs.

Seated Upper Body Exercises

Additionally, this guide also introduces a series of seated upper body exercises since it acknowledges that some seniors may prefer or require seated workouts due, to mobility limitations they might have. Seated exercises are beneficial not, for stability but for targeting important muscle groups such as the arms, shoulders, and upper back. Seniors can follow instructions to maintain posture and hand positions while performing these exercises. This ensures that each movement is precise and maximizes the benefits while minimizing the risk of strain. Let's take a look at some examples of "Seated Upper Body Exercises" specifically designed for seniors using resistance bands.

Seated Bicep Curls

Sit comfortably with a straight back and secure the resistance band under both feet.

Hold the ends of the band in each hand with palms facing forward.

Keeping your elbows close to your sides, exhale as you curl your hands towards your shoulders.

Inhale as you slowly lower your hands back to the starting position. Repeat for a set of 10-15 repetitions.

Seated Shoulder Press

Sit with the resistance band under both feet and hold the ends of the band at shoulder height.

Palms should be facing forward, and elbows bent at a 90-degree angle.

Exhale as you press the band overhead, extending your arms.

Inhale as you lower your arms back to the starting position.

Repeat for a set of 10-12 repetitions.

Seated Row

Secure the band around a sturdy post or use a door anchor at chest height.

Sit with your legs extended, wrapping the band around the soles of your feet.

Hold the ends of the band with both hands, palms facing each other.

Exhale as you pull the band towards your chest, squeezing your shoulder blades.

Inhale as you release the tension and extend your arms. Repeat for a set of 12-15 repetitions.

Seated Lateral Raises

Sit with the band under both feet and hold the ends with palms facing your body.

Keep a slight bend in your elbows and exhale as you lift your arms out to the sides.

Inhale as you lower your arms back down. Focus on controlled movements. Repeat for a set of 12-15 repetitions.

Seated Tricep Extensions

Sit with the band secured under one foot.

Hold one end of the band with both hands overhead.

Exhale as you extend your arms, lifting the band overhead.

Inhale as you bend your elbows, bringing your hands back behind your head. Repeat for a set of 10-12 repetitions.

Seated Chest Press

Sit tall with the band secured behind you around a stable post.

Hold the ends of the band in each hand, starting with your hands near your chest.
Exhale as you push the band forward, extending your arms.
Inhale as you bring your hands back towards your chest. Repeat for a set of 12-15 repetitions.

Seated Twist with Resistance
Sit with the band secured under one foot and hold the ends with both hands.
Exhale as you twist your upper body to one side, engaging your core.
Inhale as you return to the center. Repeat the twist on the other side. Alternate for a set of 10 twists on each side.

Seated Wrist Flexor and Extensor Stretch
Sit with the band secured under one foot.
Hold one end of the band with your hand, palm facing down, and gently pull for a wrist flexor stretch.
Rotate your hand, palm facing up, and pull for a wrist extensor stretch. Hold each stretch for 15-20 seconds.
the tension and extend your arms. Repeat this for a set of 12 to 15 repetitions.

These seated upper body exercises offer a workout that targets areas including arms, shoulders, chest, and back. They are designed to be gentle, effective, and adaptable, to fitness levels making them perfect for individuals who want to incorporate resistance band training into their exercise routine. Prioritize maintaining form and consult with a healthcare professional before starting any new exercise program.

Standing Upper Body Exercises

These exercises aim to improve stability and engage core muscles. Provide a workout experience. From bicep curls to raises each exercise comes with instructions on body alignment, posture, and breathing techniques. This holistic approach ensures resistance band training specifically designed for seniors.

Here are some examples of "Standing Upper Body Exercises" tailored for seniors in the context of "Resistance Band Training for Seniors".

Standing Bicep Curls

Starting Position: Stand with feet hip-width apart, securing the resistance band under both feet.

Exercise: Hold the ends of the band with palms facing forward, exhale as you curl your hands towards your shoulders, and inhale as you lower them back down. Engage your core for stability.

Benefit: Strengthens the biceps and forearms, promoting overall arm functionality.

Overhead Shoulder Press

Starting Position: Stand with one foot on the center of the resistance band, holding the ends at shoulder height.

Exercise: Exhale as you press the band overhead, extending your arms. Inhale as you bring your hands back down to shoulder height.

Benefit: Targets the shoulders and upper back, enhancing shoulder strength and stability.

Lateral Raises

Starting Position: Stand with the resistance band under both feet, holding the ends with palms facing your body.

Exercise: Exhale as you lift your arms out to the sides, keeping a slight bend in your elbows. Inhale as you lower them back down.

Benefit: Works the deltoids and improves shoulder flexibility, contributing to overall upper body tone.

Standing Tricep Extensions

Starting Position: Stand with one foot on the resistance band, holding one end with both hands overhead.

Exercise: Exhale as you extend your arms overhead, engaging the triceps. Inhale as you bend your elbows, bringing your hands back behind your head.

Benefit: Targets the triceps and improves arm strength and definition.

Standing Chest Press

Starting Position: Secure the resistance band around a stable post, standing with your back to it. Hold the ends in each hand near your chest.

Exercise: Exhale as you push the band forward, extending your arms. Inhale as you bring your hands back towards your chest.

Benefit: Strengthens the chest, shoulders, and arms, contributing to overall upper-body muscle balance.

Upright Rows

Starting Position: Stand with the resistance band under both feet, holding the ends with palms facing your body.

Exercise: Exhale as you lift the band towards your chest, keeping your elbows higher than your hands. Inhale as you lower it back down.

Benefit: Targets the muscles in the upper back and shoulders, enhancing posture.

Front Raises

Starting Position: Stand with the resistance band under both feet, holding the ends with palms facing your body.
Exercise: Exhale as you lift the band in front of you, keeping a slight bend in your elbows. Inhale as you lower it back down.
Benefit: Focuses on the front of the shoulders, improving shoulder strength and stability.

Anti-Rotation Band Twists

Starting Position: Stand with the band anchored at chest height, holding one end with both hands.
Exercise: Exhale as you twist your upper body away from the anchor point, engaging your core. Inhale as you return to the starting position.
Benefit: Strengthens the core muscles and improves torso stability.

These upper body exercises are great, for seniors as they offer a range of movements that can help improve strength, flexibility, and overall functionality of the body. It's important to focus on form starting with a level of resistance and gradually increasing intensity based on individual fitness levels.

Bicep Curls

When it comes to "Resistance Band Training for Seniors " the chapter on bicep curls is a way to build arms and improve overall upper body function. Bicep curls may seem simple. They play a role in our tailored variations designed specifically for seniors. Whether you prefer seated exercises that prioritize stability or standing exercises that also work on balance training we have carefully crafted these variations to suit fitness levels. This section not only explains how engaging the biceps affects our anatomy but also emphasizes the importance of form, breathing techniques, and gradual progression. Whether you're a fitness enthusiast or just starting your wellness journey this chapter invites seniors to experience the benefits of resistance band training, for sculpting arm strength with gentle precision.

Get ready to lift both your spirits and weights as we embark on this rejuvenating exploration of bicep curls tailored to enhance vitality and well-being in seniors.

Here are some examples of bicep exercises specifically designed for adults, as part of their resistance band training.

Seated Resistance Band Bicep Curls
Starting Position: Sit on a sturdy chair with good posture, securing the resistance band under both feet.
Exercise: Hold the ends of the band with palms facing forward. Exhale as you curl your hands towards your shoulders, engaging the biceps. Inhale as you lower them back down.
Benefit: This seated variation provides stability and targets the biceps effectively while being gentle on the lower back.

Standing Resistance Band Bicep Curls
Starting Position: Stand with feet hip-width apart, placing one foot on the center of the resistance band.
Exercise: Hold the ends with palms facing forward. Exhale as you curl your hands towards your shoulders, keeping your elbows close to your sides. Inhale as you lower them back down.
Benefit: Targets the biceps and engages core muscles for stability. The standing position adds an element of balance training.

Alternating Arm Resistance Band Bicep Curls

Starting Position: Stand or sit with good posture, securing the resistance band under both feet.

Exercise: Hold the ends of the band with palms facing forward. Exhale as you curl one hand towards your shoulder while keeping the other arm extended. Inhale as you switch arms.

Benefit: This variation adds a dynamic element, engaging both arms alternately and enhancing overall muscle coordination.

Cross-Body Resistance Band Bicep Curls

Starting Position: Stand or sit with good posture, securing the resistance band under both feet.

Exercise: Hold the ends of the band with palms facing forward. Exhale as you curl one hand diagonally across your body towards the opposite shoulder. Inhale as you lower it back down.

Benefit: Targets the biceps from a different angle, providing variation and additional engagement of the forearm muscles.

Single-Arm Resistance Band Bicep Curls

Starting Position: Stand or sit with good posture, securing the resistance band under one foot.

Exercise: Hold one end of the band with the palm facing forward. Exhale as you curl your hand towards your shoulder. Inhale as you lower it back down.

Benefit: Focuses on one arm at a time, allowing for concentrated effort and isolation of the bicep muscles.

Isometric Resistance Band Bicep Curls

Starting Position: Stand or sit with good posture, securing the resistance band under both feet.

Exercise: Hold the ends of the band with palms facing forward. Instead of a full range of motion, maintain a static hold at the midpoint of the curl for 10-15 seconds. Release and repeat.

Benefit: Introduces an isometric component, building strength in the biceps and promoting muscular endurance.

These bicep curl variations cater to seniors' diverse needs, allowing for seated or standing positions and providing options for targeting different parts of the bicep muscles. Always encourage proper form and start with a comfortable resistance level, gradually progressing as strength improves.

Shoulder Press

In the book "Resistance Band Training, for Seniors " the chapter dedicated to shoulder press offers an exploration of strengthening the body with elegance and precision. The shoulder press exercise, which holds a place in this guide is tailored to suit the specific needs of seniors. Whether performed while standing or sitting various selected versions of this exercise not only target the deltoids and trapezius muscles but also emphasize essential aspects such as maintaining good posture, controlled breathing, and gradual progression.

This section encourages seniors to delve into the art of shoulder press opportunities for better posture, enhanced shoulder stability, and a renewed sense of vigor in their upper body. As we embark on this uplifting journey the chapter on shoulder press emerges as a guiding light that promises an experience, in resistance band training aligned with the unique fitness paths seniors may follow. Prepare yourself to enhance your body strength while embracing the empowering benefits that shoulder press exercises bring to your overall well-being adventure. Here are some examples of shoulder press exercises designed specifically for seniors in the context of "Resistance Band Training for Seniors".

Seated Shoulder Press

Starting Position: Sit on a stable chair with good posture, securing the resistance band under both feet.

Exercise: Hold the ends of the band at shoulder height with palms facing forward. Exhale as you press the band overhead, extending your arms. Inhale as you lower the band back to shoulder height.

Benefit: This seated variation provides stability, targeting the shoulders and upper back while minimizing strain on the lower back.

Standing Shoulder Press

Starting Position: Stand with feet hip-width apart, placing one foot on the center of the resistance band.

Exercise: Hold the ends of the band at shoulder height with palms facing forward. Exhale as you press the band overhead, extending your arms. Inhale as you lower the band back to shoulder height.

Benefit: Engages core muscles for stability and strengthens the shoulders, trapezius, and upper back. Incorporates balance training.

Alternating Arm Shoulder Press

Starting Position: Stand with good posture, securing the resistance band under both feet.

Exercise: Hold the ends of the band with palms facing forward. Exhale as you press one arm overhead while keeping the other arm at shoulder height. Inhale as you switch arms.

Benefit: Engages both arms alternately, promoting balanced muscle development in the shoulders and upper back.

Front Shoulder Press
Starting Position: Stand with feet hip-width apart, securing the resistance band under both feet.
Exercise: Hold the ends of the band with palms facing your body. Exhale as you press the band forward, extending your arms. Inhale as you bring the band back towards your chest.
Benefit: Targets the front of the shoulders and chest, enhancing overall upper body strength and posture.

Seated Alternating Shoulder Press
Starting Position: Sit on a stable chair, securing the resistance band under both feet.
Exercise: Hold the ends of the band with palms facing forward. Exhale as you press one arm overhead while keeping the other arm at shoulder height. Inhale as you switch arms.
Benefit: Provides a seated alternative to engage the shoulders and upper back with a focus on alternating arm movements.

Diagonal Shoulder Press
Starting Position: Stand with feet hip-width apart, securing the resistance band under both feet.
Exercise: Hold the ends of the band with one hand at shoulder height and the other hand diagonally across your body. Exhale as you press the band diagonally overhead. Inhale as you return to the starting position.
Benefit: Targets the shoulders from a diagonal angle, promoting a well-rounded shoulder workout.

These shoulder press variations offer seniors a diverse range of exercises to strengthen and tone the shoulders, trapezius, and upper back. Always prioritize proper form, start with a comfortable resistance level, and progress gradually based on individual fitness levels.

Chest Press

The chapter, on chest press in the narrative "Resistance Band Training for Seniors" is an exploration of strengthening the body with care and precision. This tailored guide emphasizes variations of the chest press exercise specifically designed for seniors whether they are seated or standing. Each version focuses not on working the chest muscles but on teaching proper form, controlled breathing, and gradually increasing intensity. This section encourages seniors to discover the art of chest press promising benefits beyond toning muscles, such as improved posture and increased resilience in the body. The chest press chapter serves as a cornerstone in this enriching journey of resistance band training providing a path to experiences that align with senior's diverse wellness goals. Get ready to cultivate your body strength, with precision and embrace the empowering advantages that come with performing chest press exercises on your unique fitness journey.

Here are examples of chest press exercises tailored for seniors in the context of "Resistance Band Training for Seniors".

Seated Resistance Band Chest Press

Starting Position: Sit comfortably on a stable chair with good posture, securing the resistance band behind you around the backrest or to a sturdy post.

Exercise: Hold the ends of the band with palms facing forward. Exhale as you push the band forward, extending your arms. Inhale as you bring the band back towards your chest.

Benefit: This seated variation provides stability and effectively targets the chest muscles.

Standing Resistance Band Chest Press

Starting Position: Stand with feet hip-width apart, placing one foot on the center of the resistance band.

Exercise: Hold the ends of the band at chest height with palms facing forward. Exhale as you press the band forward, extending your arms. Inhale as you bring the band back towards your chest.

Benefit: Engages core muscles for stability and strengthens the chest, shoulders, and arms. Incorporates balance training.

Incline Resistance Band Chest Press

Starting Position: Secure the resistance band around a stable post or anchor at chest height.

Exercise: Stand with your feet staggered, facing away from the anchor point. Hold the ends of the band with palms facing forward. Exhale as you press the band diagonally upward. Inhale as you bring the band back to the starting position.

Benefit: Targets the upper chest muscles, offering a variation to work different areas of the chest.

Decline Resistance Band Chest Press

Starting Position: Secure the resistance band around a stable post or anchor at chest height.

Exercise: Stand with your feet staggered, facing toward the anchor point. Hold the ends of the band with palms facing forward. Exhale as you press the band diagonally downward. Inhale as you bring the band back to the starting position.

Benefit: Targets the lower chest muscles, providing a well-rounded chest workout.

Alternating Arm Resistance Band Chest Press

Starting Position: Stand or sit with good posture, securing the resistance band under both feet.

Exercise: Hold the ends of the band with palms facing forward. Exhale as you press one arm forward while keeping the other arm at chest height. Inhale as you switch arms.

Benefit: Engages both arms alternately, promoting balanced muscle development in the chest and shoulders.

Single-Arm Resistance Band Chest Press

Starting Position: Stand or sit with good posture, securing the resistance band under one foot.

Exercise: Hold one end of the band with the palm facing forward. Exhale as you press the band forward. Inhale as you bring the band back towards your chest.

Benefit: Focuses on one side at a time, allowing for concentrated effort and isolation of the chest muscles.

These chest press variations offer seniors a diverse range of exercises to strengthen and tone the chest, shoulders, and arms. Always prioritize proper form, start with a comfortable resistance level, and progress gradually based on individual fitness levels.

Lower Body Exercises

The chapter, on body exercises in the narrative of "Resistance Band Training for Seniors" takes us on a transformative journey to strengthen and stabilize our bodies with a touch of grace. It is a part of this wellness guide that offers tailored variations for seniors at different fitness levels. From seated movements that focus on stability to standing exercises that incorporate balance training, this section does not engage the leg muscles. Also emphasizes proper alignment, controlled breathing, and gradual progression. As we begin this rejuvenating adventure the chapter on body exercises serves as a gateway promising mobility, better posture, and a renewed sense of vitality, in our lower bodies. Let's embrace the benefits of resistance band training as we explore these exercises designed specifically for senior's unique wellness goals. Together we w Here are examples of lower body exercises tailored for seniors in the context of "Resistance Band Training for Seniors".

Seated Leg Press

Starting Position: Sit on a stable chair with good posture, securing the resistance band under both feet.

Exercise: Extend your legs, pressing against the resistance band. Exhale as you push your legs forward. Inhale as you bend your knees, returning to the starting position.

Benefit: Strengthens the quadriceps, hamstrings, and glutes with minimal impact on the joints.

Standing Hip Abduction

Starting Position: Stand with feet hip-width apart, securing the resistance band around the ankles.

Exercise: Lift one leg out to the side against the resistance of the band, exhaling as you do so. Inhale as you lower the leg back down. Switch sides and repeat.

Benefit: Targets the hip abductors, promoting hip stability and strengthening the outer thighs.

Standing Hip Extension

Starting Position: Stand with feet hip-width apart, securing the resistance band around the ankles.

Exercise: Extend one leg backward against the resistance of the band, exhaling as you do so. Inhale as you bring the leg back to the starting position. Switch sides and repeat.

Benefit: Engages the glutes and hamstrings, contributing to improved hip strength and stability.

Seated Knee Extensions

Starting Position: Sit on a stable chair with good posture, securing the resistance band under one foot.

Exercise: Extend your knee against the resistance of the band, exhaling as you do so. Inhale as you bend your knee, returning to the starting position. Switch sides and repeat.

Benefit: Targets the quadriceps, aiding in knee strength and mobility.

Seated Leg Curl

Starting Position: Sit on a stable chair with good posture, securing the resistance band around the back of one ankle.

Exercise: Curl your leg, bringing your heel toward your glutes against the resistance of the band. Exhale as you curl. Inhale as you straighten your leg. Switch sides and repeat.

Benefit: Focuses on the hamstrings, enhancing knee flexion and strengthening the back of the thighs.

Standing Calf Raises

Starting Position: Stand with feet hip-width apart, securing the resistance band under the balls of both feet.

Exercise: Rise onto your toes against the resistance of the band, exhaling as you lift. Inhale as you lower your heels back down.

Benefit: Targets the calf muscles, aiding in ankle stability and strengthening the lower legs.

Seated Inner Thigh Press

Starting Position: Sit on a stable chair with good posture, securing the resistance band between your knees.

Exercise: Press your knees outward against the resistance of the band, exhaling as you do so. Inhale as you release the pressure.

Benefit: Engages the inner thigh muscles, promoting hip stability and strengthening the adductors.

Lateral Band Walk
Starting Position: Stand with feet hip-width apart, securing the resistance band around the ankles.
Exercise: Take sideways steps against the resistance of the band, maintaining tension. Exhale with each step. Inhale as you return to the starting position.
Benefit: Targets the hips and outer thighs, enhancing lateral stability and leg strength.

These lower body exercises provide seniors with a well-rounded approach to strengthening and toning the muscles in the legs, hips, and lower body. Always prioritize proper form, start with a comfortable resistance level, and progress gradually based on individual fitness levels.

Core Strengthening Exercises

Within the realm of "Resistance Band Training, for Seniors " lies a chapter dedicated to core strengthening exercises that unveils a voyage towards cultivating stability and vitality through deliberate movements. These core exercises take stage in this wellness guide offering carefully crafted variations tailored to suit the diverse fitness levels of seniors. Whether performed in seated or standing positions each exercise does not target abdominal muscle strengthening. Also emphasizes the importance of maintaining proper posture, controlled breathing, and gradual progression. This section encourages seniors to delve into the art of core strengthening promising an array of benefits that go beyond toning muscles, including balance, enhanced support for the spinal column, and an overall sense of resilience at the core. As we embark on this empowering journey let us embrace the experiences that lie within the chapter on core strengthening exercises—a gateway to reaching wellness goals through resistance band training..

Relish, the invigorating advantages offered by these exercises as they lay a foundation of stability and vitality throughout your entire fitness endeavor.

Here are examples of core strengthening exercises tailored for seniors in the context of "Resistance Band Training for Seniors".

Seated Russian Twists

Starting Position: Sit on a stable chair with good posture, securing the resistance band around your midsection.

Exercise: Hold the ends of the band with both hands and rotate your torso to one side, feeling the resistance of the band. Return to the center and then rotate to the other side. Exhale during the twist and inhale as you return to the center.

Benefit: Engages the obliques and promotes spinal mobility.

Standing Woodchops

Starting Position: Stand with feet hip-width apart, securing the resistance band to a stable anchor at chest height.

Exercise: Hold the band with both hands and with a slight bend in your knees, rotate your torso, and lift the band diagonally across your body. Exhale during the lift and inhale as you return to the starting position.

Benefit: Targets the obliques and improves rotational strength.

Seated Leg Lifts

Starting Position: Sit on a stable chair with good posture, securing the resistance band around your midsection.

Exercise: Hold the ends of the band with both hands and lift one or both legs against the resistance of the band. Exhale during the lift and inhale as you lower the legs.

Benefit: Activates the lower abdominal muscles and enhances core stability.

Standing Pallof Press

Starting Position: Stand with feet shoulder-width apart, securing the resistance band to a stable anchor at chest height.

Exercise: Hold the band with both hands in front of your chest and press it straight out, resisting the pull of the band. Exhale during the press and inhale as you return to the starting position.

Benefit: Targets the core muscles, especially the obliques, and improves overall stability.

Seated Bicycle Crunches

Starting Position: Sit on a stable chair with good posture, securing the resistance band around your midsection.

Exercise: Hold the ends of the band with both hands and perform bicycle crunches by lifting one knee toward your chest while simultaneously twisting your torso to bring the opposite elbow towards the knee. Exhale during the crunch and inhale as you return to the starting position.

Benefit: Engages both the upper and lower abdominal muscles, promoting core strength and flexibility.

Bird Dogs with Band Resistance

Starting Position: Kneel on all fours, securing the resistance band around the bottoms of both feet.

Exercise: Lift and extend one arm and the opposite leg against the resistance of the band, creating a straight line from your fingertips to your toes. Exhale during the extension and inhale as you return to the starting position. Switch sides and repeat.

Benefit: Activates the entire core, including the lower back and glutes, promoting balance and stability.

Plank with Band Row

Starting Position: Get into a plank position with the resistance band secured under your hands.

Exercise: Perform a row by pulling one elbow towards your hip against the resistance of the band. Exhale during the row and inhale as you return to the plank position. Switch sides and repeat.
Benefit: Engages the core, especially the muscles around the mid-back, promoting strength and stability.

These core strengthening exercises offer seniors a comprehensive approach to fortifying the abdominal and back muscles, contributing to improved stability, balance, and overall core vitality. Always prioritize proper form, start with a comfortable resistance level, and progress gradually based on individual fitness levels.

Chapter 5: Progressive Workouts

In the captivating storyline of "Resistance Band Training, for Seniors " the section on workouts shines as a guiding light leading individuals through meaningful steps towards improved fitness levels. Gradual workouts, a component of this wellness guide act as a roadmap for seniors to gradually enhance their strength, flexibility, and overall well-being. These customized workouts cater to fitness levels. Follow a well-thought-out progression that builds upon past accomplishments ensuring steady and sustainable progress. As we embark on this empowering journey the gradual workouts section becomes a cornerstone equipping seniors with the tools and structure to witness enhancements in their resistance band training routine. From exercises to advanced variations, each step represents an achievement and promotes a sense of fulfillment and vitality. Come join us in unlocking the potential of resistance band training as we navigate through the designed path of progress that aligns with senior's unique fitness aspirations

Gradually Increasing Resistance

When it comes to "Resistance Band Training, for Seniors " one crucial aspect is gradually increasing the resistance over time. This approach takes into account the needs and abilities of seniors who are starting their fitness journey. The idea behind this principle is that progress is a process rather than an end goal making it a sustainable and rewarding way to incorporate resistance band training into the lives of older adults.

At its core increasing resistance acknowledges the value of making consistent improvements. It allows seniors, who may have fitness levels and health considerations to feel supported and empowered as they work towards their goals. Unlike a one-size-fits-all all approach this strategy ensures that each individual can tailor their fitness experience according to their challenges and celebrate the smallest achievements.

The fundamental concept is rooted in the understanding that everyone begins at a starting point in terms of fitness. Seniors come from backgrounds. Have varying levels of physical activity which requires a program that recognizes these differences. Using resistance bands as tools provides a means for facilitating this progression while remaining accessible, to all individuals.

For seniors, whether they are passionate, about fitness and want to maintain a lifestyle or are just starting their exercise journey the resistance band provides a way to get started and grow over time.

The process begins by assessing each individual's abilities. This involves determining the level of tension for the resistance band considering any existing health conditions and evaluating fitness levels. By finding a starting point that's both comfortable and challenging seniors can establish a foundation that's not overwhelming but still allows for progress.

One of the advantages of this approach is its focus on safety. Seniors often face issues and muscle stiffness so it's important to prioritize health and gradual adaptation. By increasing resistance, the risk of overexertion or strain is minimized. This safety-oriented strategy not only helps prevent injuries but also boosts confidence and trust in the exercise routine.

As seniors become accustomed to the levels of resistance the program evolves systematically. Progressive resistance is introduced at a pace that aligns with each individual's comfort and readiness. This means making increases, in tension or intensity as they progress on their fitness journey.

This approach recognizes the importance of fitness, as a purposeful journey, rather than a quick sprint.

In addition, the idea of increasing resistance gradually is closely linked to the principles of adaptation. Our bodies regardless of age respond positively when faced with progressive challenges. By increasing resistance over time, older adults can stimulate muscle growth improve endurance, and strengthen their bodies without overwhelming them. This adaptive response is particularly crucial for seniors who want to maintain or regain muscle mass, which plays a role in health and mobility.

What's more, this approach fosters a sense of accomplishment and motivation. Seniors often face discouragement due to the misconception that age limits progress. However, by recognizing and celebrating achievements like completing a repetition or using slightly heavier resistance bands they find renewed energy and motivation. These small victories become catalysts for dedication and commitment.

The "Resistance Band Training, for Seniors" program follows the principles of resistance increase by providing workouts that offer variety. It starts with exercises focusing on mobility, flexibility, and gentle strength building before introducing more challenging variations. This thoughtful progression allows seniors to smoothly transition from beginner movements to advanced exercises as they grow stronger and more confident.

The mental and emotional aspects of the fitness journey are just as important, as the benefits. When seniors gradually increase resistance in their workouts they not only improve their well-being but also experience a sense of accomplishment overcome challenges and develop a positive relationship with exercise. This comprehensive approach recognizes the connection between our mental health promoting a feeling of success and nurturing a mindset.

To put it simply the information in "Resistance Band Training for Seniors" goes beyond lifting weights or stretching bands. It empowers seniors to embrace a lifestyle that prioritizes their health and vitality. The narrative encourages individuals to redefine what it means to age gracefully by showing that progress is not limited by age but determined by taking steps forward.

In conclusion, increasing resistance is at the core of a fitness journey that honors each senior's story. It embodies a philosophy that acknowledges progress isn't about building strength; it's also, about fostering resilience cultivating a mindset, and celebrating our body's innate ability to adapt and thrive regardless of our age.

By embracing the progress that comes with resistance band training, "Resistance Band Training, for Seniors" goes beyond being a guidebook. It becomes a trusted companion providing seniors with a pathway, to a vibrant and fulfilling life.

Introducing Variations for Continued Challenge

In the world of "Resistance Band Training, for Seniors " the idea of incorporating exercises to keep things interesting and challenging emerges as an exciting and dynamic strategy. This approach aims to take seniors on a fitness journey that goes beyond limits. The guide understands the importance of offering a range of exercises not only to keep routines engaging but also to push the body in new and meaningful ways. As seniors embark on their fitness adventure introducing variations becomes a catalyst for maintaining interest adapting well and continuously improving their well-being.

The concept of incorporating variations for the challenge is about breaking free from monotony and embracing the versatility that resistance band training offers. Like any fitness enthusiast seniors can experience plateaus or periods where progress seems stagnant. This is where the beauty of variations comes in by injecting freshness and excitement into their workout routine. By introducing movements and challenges seniors can overcome boredom. Renew their dedication to regular exercise.

Variations are not about making workouts more complex; they are, about customizing routines based on preferences addressing specific fitness goals, and accommodating unique physical abilities.

The "Resistance Band Training, for Seniors" program offers a range of exercises that cater to individuals of fitness levels. It ensures inclusivity and accessibility by providing options that resonate with each person's body and unique fitness journey.

To keep the workout challenging and interesting it's important to understand how our bodies adapt. Our bodies can adjust to stimuli making it crucial to introduce variations in our exercise routine. By doing we create a conversation between our bodies and the exercises encouraging continuous adaptation and improvement. This adaptability is especially important for seniors who may have health considerations or physical limitations.

An important advantage of incorporating variations is the targeted engagement of muscle groups. Resistance bands, which come in tension levels allow us to isolate muscles or muscle groups effectively. This targeted approach is beneficial for seniors who want to address areas of concern or strengthen muscle groups such, as the shoulders, hips, or core. By incorporating variations into their workout routine seniors can enjoy a well-rounded exercise experience.

Additionally, variations cater to the nature of fitness goalsSeniors often have objectives when it comes to their fitness, such, as improving flexibility building strength, or enhancing health. The book "Resistance Band Training for Seniors" offers a range of exercises that specifically target these goals. This allows seniors to customize their workouts based on their aspirations giving them a sense of control and purpose in their fitness journey.

Introducing variations in exercises is a concept that aligns with the principle of overload. While increasing resistance helps in building strength incorporating variations challenges the body in ways. This does not prevent progress from plateauing. Also promotes a more comprehensive and functional form of fitness. By mimicking movements, these functional exercises seamlessly integrate into senior's routines. Enhance their strength and flexibility in day-to-day activities.

Variations also play a role in addressing the well-being of seniors by including elements of balance and stability training. These aspects are crucial for preventing falls, which is a concern for seniors. Incorporating movements, changes, in body position, or single-leg exercises not only adds excitement to the workout routine but also improves proprioception and stability. Taking this approach to fitness establishes a physical foundation that is more resilient and robust.

In the book "Resistance Band Training, for Seniors " the selected variations are not just exercises, but rather essential parts of a progressive and purposeful fitness journey. Each variation serves as a stone introducing challenges while respecting the individual's current fitness level. This thoughtful selection ensures that seniors can effortlessly incorporate these variations into their workout routines fostering a sense of achievement and motivation.

We should not underestimate the benefits of introducing these variations to maintain challenges. Like any fitness enthusiast seniors thrive on the satisfaction of accomplishing goals and mastering movements. By incorporating variations we keep their minds engaged cultivating a relationship with exercise. This mental stimulation is particularly important for seniors as it contributes to their well-being and overall life satisfaction.

Moreover having a range of exercises encourages an atmosphere of playfulness and experimentation. Seniors are encouraged to explore movements discovering what feels right for their bodies and bring them joy. This exploration goes beyond considering exercise as a task; instead, it transforms it into a dynamic experience. By incorporating an element of playfulness seniors are more likely to stay dedicated to their fitness routine, in the run.

In summary, the information presented about incorporating exercises in "Resistance Band Training, for Seniors" demonstrates how a versatile and flexible fitness routine can make an impact. It signifies a shift away from repetitive workouts embracing a dynamic approach that caters to the specific requirements and goals of older individuals. By including variations this guide becomes more than a handbook; it becomes a companion, throughout seniors fitness journey empowering them to experience ongoing improvement, vitality, and enjoyable physical activity.

Tracking Your Progress

"Monitoring Your Advancement" or "Tracking Your Progress" within the context of "Resistance Band Training, for Seniors" acts as a guiding compass supporting seniors in their comprehensive and empowering fitness journey. This is crucial because it encourages seniors to go beyond metrics and embrace progress in forms. By comprehending the intricacies of improvement and establishing personalized goals they lay the groundwork for a fitness experience driven by purpose. Physiological progress tracking addresses strength, flexibility, endurance, and joint health. Meanwhile, the psychological aspects delve into building confidence celebrating accomplishments, and fostering a relationship with activity. Seniors gain empowerment by recognizing how their physical and mental well-being are interconnected thereby transforming the concept of progress into a holistic notion. Monitoring one's advancement acts as a roadmap for seniors to navigate their fitness landscapes mindfully. It allows them to celebrate victories along the way while cultivating resilience and adopting an approach, toward well-being

Chapter 6: Targeted Workouts for Common Senior Health Concerns

In the changing world of "Resistance Band Training, for Seniors" the dedicated section on "Targeted Workouts for Common Senior Health Concerns" shines as a guiding light, for wellness. This chapter takes into account the needs of seniors understanding that tailoring fitness routines can effectively address health issues and enhance overall well-being. As we embark on this part of our fitness journey the chapter serves as a resource providing exercises and valuable insights that cater to specific health considerations. From improving mobility to enhancing balance each workout is carefully crafted to empower seniors in managing and enhancing their health. Join us on this exploration of targeted workouts that go beyond approaches embracing a fitness philosophy that prioritizes individual well-being and celebrates the diverse stories of seniors striving for optimal health.

Joint Health and Flexibility

The exploration of "Resistance Band Training, for Seniors" dives into the importance of "Joint Health and Flexibility " highlighting their role in promoting overall well-being among older individuals. This chapter underscores how resistance band exercises can be transformative providing insights into health, flexibility, and their impact on the aging process. By examining the complexities, practical workouts, and holistic advantages of maintaining joint function and flexibility this content acts as a helpful guide for seniors to embrace vitality enhance mobility, and redefine aging, with resilience and strength.

The Aging Process and Joint Resilience

The content begins by delving into the process of aging. How it affects the health of our joints. It explains how joints naturally experience wear and tear highlighting the importance of taking measures to maintain their resilience. Seniors will gain insights, into the changes that occur during aging, which will help them understand why focusing on exercises that target joint health is crucial.

"The Aging Process and Joint Resilience" within the book "Resistance Band Training for Seniors" presents information that sheds light on the connection between aging and joint health. As seniors embark on this journey they will be guided toward an understanding of aging as a shared experience rather than a hindrance. They need to grasp the changes, in their joints demystifying how wear and tear affects these vital structural components. Moreover, this content introduces the concept of resilience encouraging seniors to shift their perspective and embrace their inherent strength and adaptability. Utilizing resistance band training as a catalyst, practical and adaptable exercises are provided to promote health. Seniors are motivated to embrace aging while not sustaining but enhancing their joint resilience over time.

This content serves as a guiding beacon imparting a feeling of empowerment and motivating individuals to navigate the journey of aging. It encourages them to approach it with strength and a proactive attitude, toward their health and well-being.

Importance of Joint Mobility

The section dedicated to the "Importance of Joint Mobility", in the book "Resistance Band Training for Seniors" is a guide that sheds light on how vital joint mobility is for the overall well-being of seniors. It's important to understand that having mobility not only contributes to physical agility but also plays a key role in maintaining independence in daily activities. The content takes seniors through an exploration of how joint health and functional movement are interconnected. By understanding the significance of mobility seniors can value the benefits of having well-functioning joints. Practical. Targeted resistance exercises equip seniors with tools to improve their mobility. This content aims to promote an approach, to fitness inspiring seniors to embrace the pleasure of movements, which sets them up for an active and fulfilling lifestyle as they navigate the journey of aging.

The Synergy of Flexibility and Joint Health

This article explores the connection, between maintaining flexibility and keeping our joints healthy. It serves as a guide that emphasizes how flexibility, which refers to the range of motion around our joints plays a role in joint function and overall well-being. The article enlightens seniors about the link between cultivating flexibility and reducing the risk of injuries and age-related joint problems. It also discusses exercises that can help stretch and strengthen muscles leading to flexibility and better joint mobility. By understanding how flexibility and joint health work together seniors gain knowledge and actionable steps to achieve a balance, in their lives.

Holistic Benefits of Joint Health and Flexibility Training

The information provided in the book "Resistance Band Training, for Seniors" goes beyond exercise. It offers seniors an understanding of the benefits associated with prioritizing joint health and flexibility. It's important to explore how taking care of these aspects positively impacts dimensions of well-being. Seniors should be guided in managing pain. Shown how targeted exercises can help alleviate joint discomfort and stiffness. A focus on health and flexibility also aids in preventing falls promoting stability and coordination. The book also highlights the impact, on emotional well being emphasizing how pain-free movement and improved flexibility contribute to a mindset and a sense of accomplishment. By embracing health and flexibility training as an approach seniors are encouraged to embark on a transformative journey that reaches beyond the confines of the gym fostering resilience, joy, and an overall fulfilling quality of life.

Educational Empowerment for Long-Term Wellness

The section, on "Enhancing Education for Long Term Well being" in the book "Resistance Band Training for Seniors" plays a role in guiding seniors towards a well-informed approach to their overall health. It emphasizes the significance of understanding one's limitations encouraging seniors to pay attention to their bodies and tailor resistance band exercises according to what they can handle. By promoting self-awareness seniors gain the knowledge for gradual progress in their fitness journey. The content emphasizes the importance of incorporating resistance band training into life highlighting consistency as an aspect of long-term well-being. Seniors should be aware of insights that go beyond exercise routines as this helps establish habits and a mindset that support lasting health and vitality. Through this empowerment seniors not only acquire the tools, for immediate fitness benefits but also embark on an enduring wellness journey that spans their lives.

Osteoporosis Prevention and Bone Health

The section, in the book "Resistance Band Training for Seniors" that focuses on "Osteoporosis Prevention and Bone Health" explores strategies to protect bone health specifically addressing concerns about osteoporosis in adults. This part provides an understanding of osteoporosis which is a condition characterized by weakened bones and an increased risk of fractures. It educates seniors about the factors that contribute to the loss of bone density and highlights the role that resistance band training plays in prevention. The content includes a selected range of resistance band exercises that target weight-bearing bones like those found in the spine, hips, and wrists. These exercises aim to promote bone density and strength. The emphasis is on the significance of weight-bearing and resistance exercises in reducing the impact of osteoporosis while improving bone health. By offering insights and practical exercise options this chapter empowers seniors to actively engage in resistance band training as an effective approach, to preventing osteoporosis enabling them to develop stronger and more resilient bones.

Weight-Bearing Exercises with Resistance Bands

The opening section of the book "Resistance Band Training, for Seniors" introduces readers to the world where fitness and practicality intersect, aimed at promoting long-term well-being. Within this chapter, we delve into the interconnectedness of weight-bearing exercises and resistance band training specifically focusing on how they can enhance bone health and overall strength for seniors. The narrative begins by shedding light on the role that weight-bearing activities play in maintaining bone density and preventing conditions, like osteoporosis. We then introduce seniors to the versatility and accessibility of resistance bands as tools for adding resistance to their weight-bearing exercises. This chapter serves as a guide offering a roadmap for seniors to adopt an approach to fitness that not only emphasizes immediate benefits but also highlights the long-term advantages of incorporating resistance bands into their weight-bearing routines.

Below are examples of weight-bearing exercises with resistance bands tailored for seniors.

Resistance Band Squats

Instructions: Stand with feet shoulder-width apart, placing the resistance band just above the knees. Hold onto a sturdy chair or countertop for balance. Lower your body into a squat position, keeping your back straight and knees aligned with your toes. Rise back up to the starting position, engaging your quadriceps and glutes. The resistance band adds gentle tension, enhancing the effectiveness of the exercise.

Leg Press with Resistance Band

Instructions: Sit on a sturdy chair with your back straight and a resistance band looped around both feet. Extend one leg forward, pressing against the resistance band's tension. Hold the position briefly before returning to the starting position. This exercise targets the muscles in your thighs and helps improve lower body strength.

Standing Calf Raises with Resistance Band

Instructions: Stand with the resistance band looped around the balls of your feet, holding onto a supportive surface for balance. Lift your heels off the ground, rising onto your toes. Feel the resistance band providing added challenge to your calf muscles. Lower your heels back down, completing one repetition. This exercise promotes ankle strength and calf muscle engagement.

Bent-Over Rows for Back Strength

Instructions: Sit on a chair with a resistance band secured under your feet. Hinge forward from your hips while maintaining a straight back. Grasp the resistance band handles, and pull them toward your chest, engaging your back muscles. This exercise targets the upper and middle back, supporting posture and overall back strength.

Resistance Band Hip Abduction

Instructions: While holding onto a stable surface, loop a resistance band around your ankles. Lift one leg sideways against the band's resistance, then return to the starting position. This exercise engages the hip abductor muscles, contributing to improved hip stability and balance.

Seated Leg Press

Instructions: Sit on a chair with the resistance band looped around the balls of your feet. Extend both legs forward, pressing against the resistance band. Hold the position briefly before releasing. This exercise mimics the leg press motion, targeting the quadriceps and enhancing lower body strength.

Resistance Band Deadlifts

Instructions: Stand with your feet hip-width apart, the resistance band looped under both feet and held in your hands. Hinge at your hips, keeping your back straight, and lower your upper body toward the ground. Engage your glutes and hamstrings as you return to a standing position. This exercise enhances lower back and hamstring strength.

Remember to start with a comfortable resistance level and gradually increase intensity as strength improves. Always prioritize proper form and consult with a healthcare professional before starting a new exercise routine.

Balance and Stability Drills

The opening section of the book "Resistance Band Training, for Seniors" warmly welcomes readers to a world where strength and stability intersect. This chapter highlights the significance of balance and stability for adults underlining how these elements play a crucial role in maintaining an independent and active lifestyle. As we grow older it becomes increasingly important to preserve and improve our sense of balance as it helps prevent falls and instills confidence in activities. The chapter then delves into the exploration of how resistance bands can be tools, in refining balance and stability. However, this chapter goes beyond showcasing exercises; it takes readers on a journey that empowers seniors to strengthen their foundation fostering a sense of steadiness and self-assurance with every step they take. Whether it's standing tall or overcoming challenges the subsequent pages offer purposeful and enjoyable drills that utilize the versatility of resistance bands to enhance balance, stability, and overall well-being for older adults. Here are examples of balance and stability drills using resistance bands tailored for seniors.

Single-Leg Balance with Lateral Leg Raise

Instructions: Stand on one leg, securing the resistance band under the opposite foot. Hold onto a stable surface for support if needed. Lift the non-supporting leg laterally against the resistance band, engaging your hip muscles. This exercise enhances balance and strengthens the hip abductors.

Tandem Walk with Resistance Band

Instructions: Secure the resistance band around your ankles and stand with your feet in a tandem position (one foot directly in front of the other). Take small steps forward, maintaining the tandem stance and resisting the pull of the band. This drill challenges your stability and promotes improved gait.

Seated Marching with Resistance

Instructions: Sit on a chair with the resistance band looped around both feet. Lift one knee at a time, as if marching, against the resistance of the band. This exercise promotes stability while seated and engages core muscles, supporting overall balance.

Balance Board Squats with Resistance

Instructions: Stand on a balance board with the resistance band secured under both feet. Perform squats while maintaining balance on the board, resisting the pull of the band. This drill combines lower body strengthening with the challenge of stabilizing on an uneven surface.

Clock Reaches

Instructions: Secure the resistance band around a fixed point. Stand in the center of the band and imagine a clock face around you. Reach your foot forward to noon, then to 3 o'clock, 6 o'clock, and 9 o'clock, maintaining balance with the resistance band providing gentle tension. This exercise enhances dynamic stability.

Heel-to-Toe Walk with Band Resistance

Instructions: Place the resistance band around your ankles and walk in a straight line, placing the heel of one foot directly in front of the toes of the other. The band adds resistance to each step, challenging your balance and promoting a heel-to-toe walking pattern.

Single-leg deadlift with Band Pull

Instructions: Stand on one leg, securing the resistance band under the foot of the non-supporting leg. Hinge at your hips, extend the non-supporting leg backward and simultaneously pull the resistance band toward your chest. This drill enhances stability and strengthens the posterior chain.

Balancing Bird Dog with Resistance

Instructions: Begin on hands and knees with the resistance band looped around one foot. Extend the opposite arm and leg simultaneously while resisting the pull of the band. This exercise challenges core stability and improves coordination.

These balance and stability drills, enriched by the incorporation of resistance bands, provide seniors with engaging and purposeful exercises to fortify their foundation and enhance overall stability. Always prioritize safety and gradual progression, adjusting the resistance level according to individual abilities. Consult with a healthcare professional before starting a new exercise routine.

Chapter 7: Incorporating Cardiovascular Exercise with Resistance Bands

The beginning of the content called "Incorporating Exercise with Resistance Bands" in the book "Resistance Band Training, for Seniors" introduces readers to a combination of strength and endurance. This chapter emphasizes how important cardiovascular health is for seniors showing how it contributes to their energy and well-being. It explores how resistance bands can be seamlessly integrated into exercises providing seniors with a heart approach that goes beyond traditional workout routines. This section invites you to discover the invigorating fusion of strength training and cardiovascular fitness proving that increased heart rate and improved muscular endurance can work together harmoniously with these resistance bands. The following pages offer a guide, to exercises that bring vitality to workouts creating an enjoyable path for seniors to improve their cardiovascular health while enjoying the benefits of resistance band training. Here are examples of cardiovascular exercises with resistance bands tailored for seniors.

Resistance Band Marching in Place

Instructions: Secure the resistance band around your ankles and march in place, lifting your knees high against the resistance. This exercise elevates your heart rate while engaging the lower body muscles.

Standing Resistance Band Jumping Jacks

Instructions: Stand with the resistance band under the balls of your feet. Perform jumping jacks, stretching the band laterally with each jump. This exercise adds an element of resistance to the classic cardiovascular movement, engaging the entire body.

Resistance Band Side Steps

Instructions: Place the resistance band around your ankles and assume a semi-squat position. Take lateral steps to the right and then to the left against the resistance of the band. This exercise targets the hips and thighs, providing a cardiovascular challenge.

Seated Rowing with Resistance

Instructions: Sit on a chair with the resistance band secured around a fixed point. Hold the band handles and simulate a rowing motion, engaging your arms and back muscles. This seated cardio exercise promotes heart health while focusing on upper body strength.

Resistance Band High Knees

Instructions: Stand with the resistance band secured around a fixed point at chest height. Perform high knees against the resistance, lifting your knees as high as comfortable. This exercise enhances cardiovascular endurance and strengthens the core.

Resistance Band Stationary Bike Simulation

Instructions: Sit on a chair with the resistance band looped around your feet. Mimic a cycling motion against the resistance, engaging both your lower and upper body. This exercise provides a cardiovascular workout while seated.

Resistance Band Butt Kicks

Instructions: Stand with the resistance band around your ankles and kick your heels up towards your buttocks. This dynamic movement engages the hamstrings and elevates the heart rate, contributing to cardiovascular fitness.

Resistance Band Punches

Instructions: Stand with the resistance band secured around a fixed point. Perform punching motions, alternating arms, and maintaining a brisk pace. This exercise incorporates upper body movement and cardiovascular intensity.

Resistance Band Lateral Jumps

Instructions: Secure the resistance band around your ankles and perform lateral jumps, moving side to side. The resistance band adds challenge to the leg muscles and elevates the cardiovascular intensity.

Resistance Band Circuit Training

Instructions: Create a circuit incorporating various resistance band exercises such as squats, lunges, and rows. Perform each exercise for a set duration, moving from one to the next with minimal rest. This dynamic circuit provides both strength training and cardiovascular benefits.

These examples showcase how resistance bands can be seamlessly integrated into cardiovascular exercises, offering seniors a diverse range of options to boost their heart health and overall fitness. As always, tailor the intensity to individual capabilities and consult with a healthcare professional before starting a new exercise routine.

Low-Impact Cardio Workouts

The book "Resistance Band Training, for Seniors" highlights the significance of incorporating low-impact cardio workouts into the fitness routine of individuals. These exercises are essential for promoting health while minimizing strain on joints and reducing the likelihood of injury. Low-impact exercises are specifically designed to be gentle on the joints making them highly advantageous for seniors dealing with age-related concerns such as arthritis or joint discomfort. This approach. Caters to the needs of older adults by boosting heart health without subjecting their bodies to the high-impact forces associated with traditional cardio workouts. By utilizing resistance bands during low-impact cardio exercises seniors can add a level of resistance that helps engage muscles without placing excessive stress on their bodies like running or high-intensity aerobics do. These exercises contribute significantly to blood circulation improved endurance and overall cardiovascular fitness – all crucial elements in maintaining a healthy lifestyle as people age. Embracing low-impact cardio workouts with resistance bands allows seniors to prioritize heart health reap the benefits of activity and reduce the risk of injuries – all while fostering a well-rounded and sustainable approach, to fitness.

Interval Training for Seniors

The significance of interval training, for adults as outlined in the book "Resistance Band Training for Seniors " lies in its ability to effectively enhance fitness boost metabolism, and improve overall well-being while considering the unique needs and circumstances of seniors. Interval training involves alternating between bursts of intense exercise and periods of lower-intensity activity or rest. This approach offers advantages for seniors. Firstly interval training is time efficient making it feasible for individuals with fitness levels and busy schedules. Secondly, it can be customized to accommodate fitness levels allowing seniors to gradually increase the intensity as their endurance improves. Incorporating resistance bands into interval training further enhances its effectiveness by providing varying levels of resistance which engages muscles and promotes strength development. Additionally, studies have shown that interval training has effects on heart health blood pressure regulation, and glucose metabolism. For seniors, this can lead to improved endurance, better weight management, and overall metabolic health. The strategic use of intervals, in training allows seniors to challenge themselves while ensuring that workouts remain adaptable and safe. This approach fosters a sense of achievement boosts energy levels and contributes to maintaining a fulfilling lifestyle. The book highlights how interval training, with resistance bands, can greatly benefit seniors by offering a customized fitness strategy that suits their needs and goals. Moreover, interval training has an impact on the health of seniors. Research indicates that engaging in interval training can enhance function and memory which are crucial for overall well-being, especially as individuals age. Additionally, interval training with resistance bands provides a range of exercises that accommodate fitness levels and personal preferences. Seniors can personalize their workouts by incorporating resistance band exercises and intervals to target muscle groups promoting overall strength throughout the body. Recognizing the versatility and effectiveness of interval training in fitness the book "Resistance Band Training for Seniors" guides seniors on incorporating intervals, into their workouts using resistance bands. This empowers them to enjoy stimulating and effective workout routines aligned with their health objectives. Emphasizing the importance of interval training not only enhances health but also reinforces the idea that fitness can be enjoyable, adaptable, and tailored to individual capabilities. Making it a sustainable and fulfilling aspect of the senior lifestyle.

Chapter 8: Partner and Group Exercises

The opening section of the book "Resistance Band Training, for Seniors" provides a captivating exploration into the reasons why engaging in fitness activities with others is important. It goes beyond the approach of exercising and recognizes how partnering up or participating in group exercises can greatly impact senior's overall well-being.

The chapter delves into the emotional and physical advantages of sharing the fitness journey highlighting the benefits that arise when incorporating resistance bands into collaborative workouts. By fostering connections, accountability, and mutual support, partner and group exercises not only promote physical health but also create vibrant spaces for social interaction and motivation.

This section sets the stage for seniors to collectively explore resistance band training inviting them to discover the delight of shared wellness and reinforcing the idea that fitness is not an individual pursuit but a dynamic and uplifting community endeavor. The significance of Partner and Group Exercises in "Resistance Band Training for Seniors" goes beyond notions of workout routines. It represents an exploration, into well-being acknowledging that exercise offers benefits that extend beyond just physical aspects.

This chapter demonstrates the impact that shared experiences can have on senior's overall well-being particularly when it comes to partner and group exercises. The true significance of engaging in exercises with a partner or, within a group lies in the creation of a motivating environment. Seniors often face challenges on their fitness journeys, such as limitations or a lack of motivation.

However, by participating in exercises, these challenges are met with a spirit that encourages and holds each other accountable. The shared commitment to wellness becomes a driving force bringing purpose and consistency to senior's fitness routines. The psychological benefits of exercise are deeply rooted in our need for connection and social interaction. During the years when social circles may change and external pressures mount group exercises go beyond just physical activity – they serve as a lifeline for social connection. The bonds formed during these moments of exertion create a network that reduces feelings of isolation and enhances well-being. Incorporating resistance bands, into these shared workouts serves as an element connecting individuals through their pursuit of fitness goals. Resistance band training is highly adaptable and suitable, for individuals of all fitness levels and abilities making it particularly valuable for Partner and Group Exercises aimed at seniors.

Regardless of differences in strength, flexibility, or mobility resistance bands provide a platform that allows everyone to actively participate. Within this chapter, you will find a range of exercises designed to promote inclusivity within the fitness community. These exercises include partner-assisted stretches synchronized resistance band movements and collaborative circuit training carefully selected to cater to needs. Apart from the benefits these exercises also foster an uplifting atmosphere by encouraging communal participation. The shared sense of accomplishment derived from achieving goals the moments of laughter during challenging moments and the collective celebration of progress all contribute to an enhanced fitness experience.

This emphasis on Partner and Group Exercises extends beyond well-being and taps into our human desire for connection, camaraderie, and mutual achievements. Moreover engaging in workouts affects seniors as they witness firsthand the dedication and progress made by their exercise partners. This serves as a motivator for them to stay committed, to their fitness goals. The bonds formed during these shared moments establish a feeling of responsibility, where each participant becomes a part of the effort to improve one's health. Incorporating resistance bands, into partner and group exercises brings an added layer of engagement. These bands serve not only as tools for resistance but also as a unifying force that strengthens the sense of connection. When individuals work together pulling against the resistance their combined effort becomes a symbol of the spirit within the group. The versatility of resistance bands ensures that each participant can adjust the intensity according to their abilities promoting a sense of independence and empowerment in their fitness journey To summarize Partner and Group Exercises enhanced by incorporating resistance bands play a role in creating a comprehensive and empowering fitness community for seniors. This section pays tribute to the physical aspects of exercise by portraying it as more than just an individual task— it is a shared celebration of well-being. As you continue reading through these pages you'll be encouraged to embrace the joy of exercising with others while reinforcing the idea that using resistance bands as tools transforms your quest, for better health into a collective and uplifting adventure.

Social Benefits of Group Workouts

The section, in the book "Resistance Band Training for Seniors" that talks about the "Social Benefits of Group Workouts" explores the advantages that seniors can experience when they come together to engage in fitness activities using resistance bands. It goes beyond exercise and delves into how group workouts can positively impact senior's social and emotional well-being. At its core group workouts provide a platform for interaction and connection. When individuals unite with a shared goal of improving their health a sense of camaraderie naturally emerges. The content emphasizes the significance of these bonds highlighting how they contribute to creating a motivating environment. For seniors those who may face isolation or reduced social engagement group workouts become more than exercise—they become a vital way to foster meaningful connections. The narrative continues by discussing how group workouts can help combat feelings of loneliness and create a sense of belonging. As participants synchronize their movements face challenges together and celebrate victories collectively the dynamic, within the group becomes a source of support. This content underscores how these shared experiences contribute to health outcomes by promoting a sense of purpose while reducing the risk of depression or anxiety.

Furthermore, group workouts offer advantages, including accountability and motivation, within the community. Seniors tend to stay dedicated to their fitness routines when they know they have a group counting on their presence. The concept of encouragement is explored in the content highlighting how it pushes individuals beyond their limits fostering a sense of achievement and empowerment among the collective. In these group workouts, resistance bands play a role by providing a tool that brings participants together regardless of their fitness levels. The content delves into how resistance bands allow each participant to adjust the intensity according to their abilities while still being a part of the effort. This adaptability promotes inclusivity ensuring that everyone can actively engage and benefit from the group exercise experience regardless of their condition. Moreover, the content emphasizes the enjoyment and fun that accompany group workouts in one's fitness journey. As seniors exercise with resistance bands alongside their peers it becomes more than exertion; it becomes an atmosphere filled with shared laughter, camaraderie, and joy derived from moving together as a unit. This joy serves as a motivator that makes exercise both pleasurable and sustainable, within a context. In a nutshell, the section, on "The Social Advantages of Exercising in Groups" found in the book "Resistance Band Training for Older Adults" highlights how using resistance bands can lead to experiences in terms of fitness. It goes beyond exercise and emphasizes the importance of group workouts as a way to connect socially combat feelings of loneliness foster a sense of belonging and boost mental well-being. The narrative encourages adults to embrace the aspects of staying fit and shows that by using resistance bands together they can embark on a journey, towards better health that is not only uplifting but also socially rewarding. Now let's explore further into the various ways group workouts with resistance bands can benefit seniors socially.

Shared Experience and Camaraderie

Exercising in a group setting brings people together allowing them to embark on a fitness journey, as a team. It's fascinating how this shared experience helps everyone understand each other's challenges and successes creating a sense of camaraderie. Seniors who participate in resistance band exercises alongside their peers often find solace and motivation knowing that they have companions on the path, toward health.

Combating Loneliness

The story emphasizes the importance of group exercise, as a way to combat loneliness, which is a worry, among older adults. When people take part in group workouts they have the chance to make connections exchange stories and form friendships. The feeling of belonging that comes from these interactions creates a support system that goes beyond exercising together.

Emotional Support and Mental Well-Being

Apart, from the elements the content delves into the benefits of group workouts. When individuals share their fitness goals celebrate accomplishments and encourage one another the group becomes a source of reinforcement. This sense of support plays a role, in enhancing mental well being alleviating stress, and cultivating a sense of purpose.

Mutual Encouragement and Motivation

Group exercise sessions flourish due, to the support and motivation provided by participants. This article explores how the interactions within a group can inspire and drive individuals toward their fitness objectives. When people observe the determination and advancements made by their peers it serves as an incentive for them to stay dedicated, to their health goals. The shared pursuit of wellness transforms into a voyage of development and accomplishment.

Accountability and Consistency

The content emphasizes the role of accountability within a group setting. Seniors are more likely to stick to their fitness routines when they feel a sense of responsibility to the group. The scheduled group workouts create a routine that enhances consistency, a crucial factor in realizing long-term health benefits.

Inclusivity through Adaptability

Resistance bands contribute to the inclusivity of group workouts by offering adaptability. The content explores how these bands cater to various fitness levels and physical abilities. Participants can adjust the resistance to match their capabilities, ensuring that everyone, regardless of their starting point, can actively engage in the exercises. This adaptability fosters a supportive and non-judgmental environment.

Enjoyment and Fun

Group workouts offer more, than exercise; they provide a dimension that adds enjoyment and fun. This content recognizes the significance of laughter. Shared joy during these sessions. When seniors participate in resistance band exercises the atmosphere becomes lively and engaging making the fitness journey not only beneficial but genuinely enjoyable.

To summarize group workouts using resistance bands for seniors go beyond benefits. This content highlights how these collective fitness experiences foster a sense of community, combat loneliness offer support, and create an environment where seniors can thrive not only physically but also socially and emotionally. It encourages seniors to embrace the aspects of fitness by emphasizing that with resistance bands, as tools the pursuit of better health can become a shared and uplifting adventure.

Safe and Effective Partner Exercises

The content on "Safe and Effective Partner Exercises" in the book "Resistance Band Training for Seniors" delves into a comprehensive guide designed to ensure that seniors can engage in partner workouts with the utmost safety and effectiveness. It recognizes that safety is paramount, particularly for seniors who may have varying levels of physical ability and potential health considerations.

Safety Guidelines

The content starts by outlining essential safety guidelines for partner exercises using resistance bands. This includes considerations such as proper warm-up routines, the importance of clear communication between partners, and guidelines for choosing the right resistance level based on individual capabilities. By establishing a foundation of safety protocols, seniors are empowered to embark on their partner workouts with confidence.

Joint-Friendly Movements

The narrative explores partner exercises that prioritize joint-friendly movements. It acknowledges that seniors may have joint-related concerns, and therefore, the chosen exercises are designed to be gentle on the joints while still providing effective resistance. The content highlights the importance of fluid and controlled movements to reduce the risk of injury.

Gradual Progression

Understanding that seniors may have varying fitness levels, the content emphasizes the concept of gradual progression. It provides a structured approach to increasing the intensity of partner exercises over time. This ensures that seniors can adapt to the exercises at their own pace, fostering a sense of accomplishment and minimizing the risk of overexertion.

Assistance and Support

The content demonstrates partner exercises that involve one partner providing assistance or support to the other. This might include assisted stretching or exercises where one partner helps stabilize the other. The emphasis is on the supportive nature of these exercises, promoting mutual assistance while prioritizing the safety of both individuals involved.

Adaptability to Individual Needs

Recognizing that each senior may have unique needs and considerations, the content guides how partner exercises can be adapted to accommodate individual requirements. Whether adjusting the resistance level, modifying the range of motion, or incorporating additional support, the aim is to make partner exercises accessible and beneficial for all seniors.

Communication and Feedback

Effective communication between workout partners is a key theme throughout the content. It stresses the importance of open communication to ensure that both individuals feel comfortable and safe during the exercises. Additionally, the narrative encourages partners to provide feedback to each other, fostering a collaborative and supportive atmosphere.

Versatility of Resistance Bands

The content explores how the versatility of resistance bands enhances the safety and effectiveness of partner exercises. Resistance bands provide a controlled and adaptable form of resistance, making them suitable for a wide range of movements. The narrative illustrates how these bands can be incorporated into partner exercises to target different muscle groups while minimizing the risk of strain.

In summary, "Safe and Effective Partner Exercises" serves as a comprehensive resource within the book "Resistance Band Training for Seniors." It not only introduces a variety of partner exercises tailored for safety but also emphasizes the importance of clear communication, gradual progression, and adaptability to individual needs. By focusing on these principles, the content ensures that seniors can engage in partner workouts with confidence, fostering a positive and empowering experience in their fitness journey.

Chapter 9: Setting Realistic Goals

Starting a fitness journey designed for adults shows a strong commitment, to well-being. The beginning of the chapter on "Setting Realistic Goals" in the book "Resistance Band Training for Seniors" sets an energizing tone that lays the foundation for a long-lasting experience. It acknowledges that motivation is like a spark, fueled by goals and the desire for vitality. This section addresses the obstacles that seniors might face and offers strategies not only for getting started but also for maintaining enthusiasm along the way. As we explore the relationship between motivation and consistency we realize that resistance bands are not just exercise tools; they become companions on our journey toward health. This introduction encourages adults to see their fitness pursuit as a lifestyle rather than a temporary effort, where each resistance band exercise contributes to a vibrant, consistent, and rewarding path toward well-being.

As we delve into the exploration of motivation and consistency we discover how resistance bands have an impact beyond exercise. The narrative inspires adults to approach their fitness journey with resilience understanding that challenges are stepping stones, toward lasting success.

It promotes a mentality that prioritizes progress of striving for perfection. It recognizes that achieving results is a process filled with small victories, along the way. Additionally, the introduction highlights the importance of building a community, where individuals can draw strength from shared experiences and receive encouragement, from minded people. As we delve into this section our main objective becomes clear; to inspire and empower seniors not just to begin their resistance band training but to maintain an enduring dedication to their well-being. This will create a blend of motivation, regularity, and lifelong vitality.

The Importance of Setting Realistic Goals

This content on "Setting Realistic Goals" in the book "Resistance Band Training for Seniors" is a thoughtful guide designed to help seniors navigate their fitness journey with purpose and attainable objectives. Recognizing the diversity of seniors' experiences, abilities, and aspirations, this section offers a tailored approach to goal-setting, promoting not only physical well-being but also a positive and sustainable mindset.

Understanding Individual Needs

The content starts by highlighting the importance of recognizing the needs and abilities of seniors. It encourages an approach, to setting goals considering the health backgrounds and fitness levels that seniors may have. By understanding these factors seniors can establish goals that are both challenging and achievable leading to a sense of accomplishment. In the book "Resistance Band Training for Seniors " the section on "Understanding Needs" delves into the concept of acknowledging and respecting the distinct characteristics, abilities, and situations of each senior embarking on their fitness journey. It emphasizes that a one-size-fits-all approach is not appropriate for seniors due to their health backgrounds, fitness levels, and aspirations. This section motivates seniors to take an introspective approach to their well-being. It encourages them to understand their limitations, strengths, and objectives. By doing seniors can set meaningful goals that align with their current level of fitness. This ensures that their resistance band training is tailored to meet their needs. The narrative emphasizes that fitness is a journey and this content serves as a guide, for seniors as they navigate this path according to their circumstances. It emphasizes the importance of appreciating where individuals begin their fitness journey whether they are experienced fitness enthusiasts or new to exercise. Taking into account needs also involves considering factors, beyond abilities like existing health conditions, personal preferences, and lifestyle choices. The content encourages seniors to reflect on what aspects of their health and well-being matter most to them helping them establish goals that are not attainable but also personally meaningful. By embracing the principle of understanding needs seniors can lay a foundation for a fitness journey that is effective and enjoyable. This personalized approach ensures that resistance band training becomes a unique and empowering experience for each senior promoting a sense of fulfillment and overall well-being as they progress towards health. The content within the book "Resistance Band Training, for Seniors" goes beyond acknowledging diversity; it advocates for an understanding of the distinctive qualities that each senior brings to their fitness journey. It highlights the significance of recognizing not only capabilities but also the broader range of personal circumstances, preferences, and aspirations. This section explores the concept that fitness is a journey, which requires an understanding of where each individual begins. Whether seniors have experience, with exercise or are just starting this content encourages them to think about their starting point. By doing they can approach resistance band training with self-awareness and a realistic view of their fitness levels. Furthermore "Understanding Needs" encourages seniors to consider factors beyond the aspect. Health conditions, lifestyle preferences, and personal goals all play a role in well-being. This content guides seniors in reflecting on what matters to them. Empowers them to set goals that align not only with their physical abilities but also with their values and aspirations. In essence, this section becomes a guiding principle for seniors urging them to embrace their qualities and tailor their fitness journey accordingly. By understanding needs seniors can develop a connection, to their well-being and make resistance band training a personalized and empowering experience. This thoughtful approach guarantees that the fitness journey isn't, about adhering to a one-size-fits-all all-exercise regimen but about forging a personalized path that genuinely connects with the unique circumstances and aspirations of each senior individual.

Tailoring Goals to Fitness Levels
Seniors have levels of fitness. The content helps them customize their goals based on their current abilities. It suggests starting with targets that align, with each individual's starting point gradually advancing as strength, endurance, and flexibility improve. This approach ensures that goals remain achievable and motivating throughout the resistance band training journey.

The "Tailoring Goals to Fitness Levels" section in the book "Resistance Band Training for Seniors" explores how to create fitness objectives that perfectly match an individual's capabilities. It promotes an approach acknowledging that seniors begin their fitness journeys from points.

Of imposing benchmarks this section encourages seniors to set goals that reflect their unique fitness levels and aspirations. It recognizes that some seniors may already have experience, with exercise while others are just starting. By embracing this diversity the content creates an environment where goals are not predetermined but shaped dynamically by individuals current strengths and limitations.

The narrative highlights the importance of setting goals that are both challenging and attainable. Seniors are urged to consider exercises and resistance levels that push them beyond their comfort zones fostering growth and progress.

However, the main focus remains on setting goals that ensure fitness pursuits remain enjoyable and sustainable. Additionally the concept of "Tailoring Goals, to Fitness Levels" is introduced to emphasize progression over time. Seniors are encouraged to adjust their goals as they make improvements in strength, endurance, and flexibility. This adaptable approach guarantees that goals stay relevant, challenging, and reflective of each individual's evolving fitness journey.

Essentially this content acts as a guide for seniors when it comes to goal setting. It promotes an approach that recognizes and accommodates fitness levels fostering a sense of empowerment and accomplishment. By customizing goals based on fitness levels, seniors can embark on a fitness journey that is meaningful to them and contributes to their long-term well-being.

The information provided in the book "Resistance Band Training for Seniors" regarding "Tailoring Goals to Fitness Levels" represents a way of setting goals by acknowledging the range of experiences and capabilities, among seniors. The narrative serves as a roadmap encouraging seniors to pursue a fitness journey tailored specifically to their abilities, aspirations, and preferences.

At its core, the concept revolves around recognizing that fitness is not a one-size-fits-all pursuit, for adults who come from diverse backgrounds and experiences when it comes to their wellness journey. This section acknowledges that some seniors may already have a foundation of fitness knowledge and routines while others may be taking their steps towards a more active lifestyle. By embracing this range of experiences the content paves the way for inclusive goal setting.

The focus on tailoring goals to fitness levels is not about conforming to a standard of achievement but rather about acknowledging and valuing each person's unique starting point. For seniors who are reintroducing themselves to exercise the emphasis is on setting goals that are realistic, attainable, and considerate of any potential challenges they may face. On the other hand for those who're more familiar with fitness routines the content encourages them to establish goals that offer an appropriate level of challenge ensuring ongoing growth and progress.

An important aspect of this narrative is the understanding that goals should be adaptable and evolve along with progress. The content introduces the concept of a journey where seniors adjust and modify their objectives as they witness improvements, in strength, endurance, and flexibility.

This approach encourages a mindset that sees fitness as an ever-changing journey discouraging expectations and allowing for a more flexible and enjoyable experience.

Furthermore the concept of "Tailoring Goals, to Fitness Levels" helps seniors find a balance between challenging themselves and setting goals. If goals are too ambitious it can lead to frustration or potential injury; whereas if they are too modest they may not provide stimulation for growth. This narrative encourages seniors to find a ground by selecting exercises and resistance levels that push them beyond their comfort zones fostering a sense of accomplishment without overwhelming them.

Throughout this exploration, the content tells a story that emphasizes the result. Also the process itself. Seniors are encouraged to appreciate the steps they take forward recognizing that each progress is worth celebrating. The focus on the journey serves as motivation reinforcing the idea that setting and achieving fitness goals is intrinsically rewarding and fulfilling.

In summary "Tailoring Goals to Fitness Levels" goes beyond goal setting; it becomes a philosophy that seniors can incorporate into their fitness journey. It invites them to see fitness through personalized lenses, adaptability, and an appreciation, for progress.

By customizing fitness objectives according to fitness levels older adults can begin a long-lasting fitness journey that not only caters, to their current abilities but also empowers them to grow and flourish.

Focusing on Functional Fitness

The article emphasizes the importance of setting goals that focus on fitness highlighting the improvements it brings to activities. Whether it's improving mobility, balance, or stamina having functional fitness goals ensures that seniors experience real-life benefits and overall well-being. The section titled "Focusing on Functional Fitness" in the book "Resistance Band Training, for Seniors" promotes a practical approach to exercise specifically designed for adults. Focusing on appearance or isolated muscle groups this part encourages seniors to set fitness goals that directly enhance their ability to perform everyday tasks and improve their overall well-being. At its core, the narrative challenges the concept of fitness by shifting the focus towards fitness. Than pursuing exercises for aesthetic purposes seniors are encouraged to set goals that align with the activities they encounter in their daily lives. This approach ensures that the advantages gained from resistance band training extend beyond gym sessions and positively impact real-world situations. The narrative introduces the idea that functional fitness encompasses a range of movements, for daily functionality. These activities include walking, reaching, bending, and lifting. These basic actions, when enhanced through resistance band exercises greatly improve the quality of life for individuals. This section also examines the concept of fitness. By focusing on exercises that replicate the movements required in life seniors can develop strength and flexibility, in areas that are prone to strain or injury. The narrative emphasizes that functional fitness goes beyond looking good; it's about building resilience fostering independence and reducing the risk of injury as one faces the challenges of aging. Moreover, the content highlights how resistance bands are tools that facilitate fitness. These versatile aids can be used to imitate movements for daily activities like lifting groceries or reaching for items on high shelves. The narrative explores how resistance bands offer a way for seniors to engage in exercises relevant to their functional needs. This narrative approach also encourages a change in mindset. Seniors are urged to view fitness not as an isolated pursuit but, as a part of their lifestyle. By aligning their fitness goals, with the activities that matter most to them such as spending time with grandchildren tending to their gardens or maintaining a life seniors can discover a greater sense of purpose and motivation through resistance band training. "Focusing on Functional Fitness" goes beyond the understanding of exercise. Creates a philosophy that encourages seniors to embrace a form of fitness that is meaningful, relevant, and directly applicable to their daily lives. By prioritizing fitness through resistance band training seniors not only improve their physical well-being but also develop a more meaningful and empowered approach to aging. The content in the book "Resistance Band Training for Seniors" explores this shift in perspective—a departure from fitness concepts, towards a holistic approach. It invites seniors to redefine their fitness goals beyond appearance. Instead focuses on how exercise can enhance their everyday activities. Ultimately this narrative challenges the belief that fitness is about sculpting muscles or achieving a specific look. Instead, it suggests a shift, towards fitness, which is based on the concept that exercises should reflect and improve the movements for everyday tasks. Seniors are encouraged to set goals that lead to enhancements in their ability to walk, bend, lift, and carry out regular activities. This approach to fitness is rooted in the belief that the advantages gained from resistance band training should extend beyond the confines of a gym setting. Seniors are urged to consider how their exercises can be applied in real-life situations establishing a connection between their fitness routine and the demands of their lives. In doing resistance band training is positioned not as a means to an end but as an integral part of a more active and engaged lifestyle. The narrative explores the implications of fitness by delving into its preventive aspects. By focusing on exercises that directly target the movements and muscle groups involved in activities seniors can enhance strength and flexibility in areas that are particularly prone to strain or injury. This preventive approach becomes vital, for maintaining independence and mitigating the risks associated with aging. Furthermore, emphasis is placed on highlighting how resistance bands can adapt effectively to enable fitness. These versatile tools serve as a way to mimic the movements needed in life making it easier for seniors to engage in exercises that directly match their functional needs. The story acts as a guide showing how resistance bands can be used to imitate tasks, like lifting groceries or reaching for items on shelves. This helps seniors understand how the exercises relate to real-life situations. Beyond the benefits, the story encourages a shift in mindset. Seniors are urged to see fitness not as something isolated but as a purposeful part of their overall lifestyle. By aligning fitness goals with activities that hold meaning, such as spending time with grandchildren tending to a garden or actively participating in activities seniors can find deeper motivation and satisfaction in their resistance band training. Ultimately "Focusing on Functional Fitness" becomes more than a concept—it becomes a narrative philosophy that guides seniors towards adopting an approach to fitness that goes beyond boundaries. It becomes a path, towards exercise that's meaningful and relevant—enhancing not physical well-being but also enriching the quality and vibrancy of daily life. The story unravels, as a guide that encourages adults to embrace fitness by using resistance bands. It aims to promote resilience, independence, and a fulfilling aging process.

Short-Term and Long-Term Objectives
Taking a perspective into account the content introduces the idea of having both term and long-term goals. Short-term goals serve as milestones, for motivation. Maintaining momentum with long-term goals provides a broader vision and sense of

purpose. This approach combines gratification with progress creating a roadmap that encompasses both aspects. In the book "Resistance Band Training for Seniors " the section on "Term and Long Term Objectives" explores the balance between achieving immediate results and striving for long-lasting aspirations. Then following milestones this section unfolds as a narrative guide that encourages seniors to embrace a dynamic approach to goal setting. It acknowledges the importance of short-term objectives as checkpoints that offer measures of progress and success. These goals do not provide a sense of accomplishment. They also, act as building blocks toward a more comprehensive fitness journey. The narrative emphasizes viewing short-term goals not as isolated achievements but as parts contributing to a fitness picture. By embracing this perspective seniors are motivated to continue their resistance band training, with enthusiasm.

At the time this content explores the idea of having long-term goals. Acknowledges that a fulfilling fitness journey goes beyond just short-term achievements. Long-term aspirations provide a vision. Help guide seniors towards sustained well-being and vitality. These goals could involve building strength improving mobility or reaching a specific fitness level that aligns with an individual's health and lifestyle objectives. The narrative emphasizes the importance of blending term and long-term objectives, into a story. Short-term accomplishments serve as stones laying the foundation for achieving significant and lasting goals. The interaction between these different time frames creates an evolving journey, fostering progress and continuity. Furthermore, this content delves into how objectives can adapt over time. As seniors progress through their resistance band training journey their goals may naturally change to align with strengths, interests, or shifting priorities. This adaptability ensures that goals remain relevant and meaningful while avoiding stagnation and maintaining a sense of purpose throughout the long-term trajectory. The narrative encourages seniors to recognize the interconnectedness, between short-term aspirations and long-term objectives. Short-term goals play a role, in keeping motivation alive by offering satisfaction while long-term objectives provide a sense of purpose and direction shaping the overall trajectory of one's fitness journey. In the context of seniors and their resistance band training, "Term and Long Term Objectives" serves as a narrative guide that encourages them to adopt a purposeful approach to goal setting. It emphasizes the importance of celebrating victories as components of their broader well-being story. By striking a balance between short-term wins and enduring aspirations seniors can cultivate fulfillment and longevity in their resistance band training journey.

The book "Resistance Band Training for Seniors" delves into the concept of "Short-Term and Long-Term Objectives" as an engaging narrative that inspires seniors to embrace flexibility in their goal-setting process. It highlights the interplay between short-term accomplishments and lasting ambitions.

The narrative begins by acknowledging the significance of short-term goals. These milestones act as checkpoints along the fitness journey offering measures of progress and success for seniors. Short-term objectives provide a sense of achievement and motivation acting as catalysts that fuel enthusiasm, for continued resistance band training. Considering these short-term goals as separate the narrative encourages seniors to see them as interconnected contributing to a more comprehensive fitness story. At the time it explores long-term objectives by emphasizing that a fulfilling fitness journey goes beyond just focusing on short-term goals. Long-term aspirations provide seniors with a vision that guides them toward well-being and vitality. These goals can include overarching themes like increasing strength improving mobility or achieving specific fitness levels based on individual health and lifestyle goals. The narrative doesn't follow a progression of goals. Delves, into the dynamic relationship between short-term and long-term objectives. Short-term successes are not endpoints in themselves; instead, they serve as stones toward accomplishments. They lay the foundation, for achieving lasting goals while creating a sense of progress and continuity throughout the fitness journey. Furthermore, the content examines how objectives can adapt over time. As seniors progress through their resistance band training journey their goals may naturally evolve. This adaptability ensures that fitness objectives remain relevant and meaningful preventing any sense of stagnation. The narrative aims to inspire seniors to appreciate how their goals evolve aligning them with their strengths, emerging interests, or changing priorities. Its essence lies in inviting seniors to recognize the interconnectedness of term and long-term objectives. Short-term goals provide satisfaction, which fuels motivation for the journey. Simultaneously long-term goals offer a sense of purpose and direction guiding the trajectory of the fitness journey. This narrative serves as a guiding philosophy that encourages a holistic perspective, on goal setting. In essence "Term and Long Term Objectives" acts as a companion narrative that urges seniors to celebrate victories while keeping their focus on the broader vision of well-being. By embracing this nuanced approach seniors can cultivate fulfillment, purpose, and longevity in their resistance band training journey. Then viewing it as a series of isolated accomplishments they see it as a changing story of lifelong vitality.

Adapting Goals Over Time

The content, of the book "Resistance Band Training for Seniors" acknowledges that the fitness journey is not fixed but rather a dynamic process. It encourages seniors to be open to adapting their goals as they progress through their resistance band training. This adaptability ensures that their goals remain meaningful and challenging fostering growth.

The section on "Adapting Goals Over Time" presents a narrative that recognizes the nature of fitness journeys for seniors. It emphasizes the importance of embracing a mindset of adaptation and evolution in setting and adjusting goals.

Of treating fitness goals as milestones this narrative introduces the concept that goals should be flexible adjusting according to a senior's progress in resistance band training. This flexibility is rooted in the understanding that individuals experience changes in fitness levels, preferences, and overall well-being over time.

The narrative highlights the significance of staying attuned to one's body and acknowledging circumstances as they change. Through engaging in resistance band training seniors may discover strengths encounter evolving health conditions or develop interests. Adapting goals becomes a way to align their fitness journey, with these shifts while ensuring objectives stay relevant and purposeful.

Moreover, this content explores the concept that adjusting goals is not a sign of weakness but an expression of self-awareness and adaptability. Older individuals are encouraged to acknowledge and celebrate progress while remaining open, to modifying their goals in response to changing circumstances. This mindset promotes a sense of empowerment enabling individuals to shape their fitness journey.

The narrative also delves into the notion that adapting goals over time contributes to an enjoyable fitness experience. It discourages overly ambitious approaches that may result in frustration or burnout. Instead, the narrative suggests that evolving goals bring about challenges and engagement making the resistance band training journey not only effective but also fulfilling and enjoyable.

Essentially "Adapting Goals Over Time" becomes a guiding principle for seniors reminding them that the path to well-being is not linear but an ever-evolving journey. The narrative encourages a flexible approach to goal setting, fostering resilience and empowerment in the face of fluctuations accompanying the aging process. By embracing the idea of adapting goals over time seniors can cultivate a lifelong commitment, to resistance band training.

In the book "Resistance Band Training, for Seniors " the section on "Adapting Goals Over Time" takes a storytelling approach to highlight how the fitness journey is always changing and evolving. It encourages seniors to embrace a mindset of adjusting their goals.

The narrative emphasizes that fitness goals shouldn't be fixed benchmarks. Instead, it suggests that seniors should see their goals as entities that can adapt and transform alongside their progress in resistance band training. This adaptability stems from recognizing that our bodies, lifestyles, and health conditions change as we age.

A key aspect of this narrative is being attuned to one's body and circumstances. As seniors engage in resistance band training they may discover strengths encounter health considerations or develop new interests. The idea of adapting goals is presented as a way to align one's fitness journey with these shifts ensuring that objectives remain relevant, meaningful, and aligned with an individual's evolving well-being.

Furthermore, the content explores the notion that adjusting goals is not a sign of weakness but an expression of self-awareness and responsiveness. Seniors are encouraged to celebrate their progress while also remaining open, to modifying their goals based on changing circumstances.

This mentality of adaptability becomes a source of strength allowing individuals to actively shape their fitness journey based on their needs and aspirations. The story further emphasizes the notion that adjusting goals over time contributes to an enjoyable fitness experience. It discourages an overly ambitious approach that may result in frustration or burnout. Instead, the narrative suggests that evolving goals create a sense of challenge and involvement. This does not make resistance band training effective. Also ensures that it remains fulfilling and enjoyable promoting a positive and lasting relationship, with physical activity.

Essentially "Adapting Goals Over Time" acts as a guiding principle that reminds adults that the path to well-being is not linear but rather a dynamic and evolving process. The narrative encourages a flexible approach to setting goals fostering resilience and empowerment in the face of changes associated with aging. By embracing the concept of adjusting goals over time older adults can cultivate a lifelong commitment, to resistance band training ensuring it remains an uplifting and enriching aspect of their overall well-being.

Celebrating Achievements

The content emphasizes the significance of celebrating accomplishments no matter how small they may be. By acknowledging and appreciating progress older individuals develop a mindset that reinforces their dedication to resistance band training. Regular recognition of achievements contributes to a sense of fulfillment. Creates a cycle of reinforcement.

In the book "Resistance Band Training, for Seniors " the section on "Celebrating Achievements" unfolds as a story that highlights the importance of acknowledging and rejoicing in the progress made throughout one's fitness journey.

At its core, this narrative encourages seniors to adopt a mindset that values both the victories and the significant milestones achieved through resistance band training. Of focusing on reaching their ultimate fitness goals the narrative invites seniors to appreciate and celebrate each step forward along their journey.

The narrative delves into the notion that celebrating achievements extends beyond outcomes. It encompasses improvements in well being increased energy levels, enhanced mood, and newfound confidence gained through exercise. By expanding what it means to achieve something this narrative encourages seniors to recognize and cherish the benefits that come from their commitment to resistance band training. Furthermore, the content underscores that celebration serves as a motivator.

By taking the time to acknowledge their accomplishments older adults create a feedback loop that reinforces their dedication to staying fit. This positive reinforcement serves as motivation leading to an enjoyable exercise routine.

Moreover, the narrative emphasizes the importance of embracing the uniqueness of each person's fitness journey. Every individual's progress is personal and distinct influenced by their starting point, goals, and the obstacles they have overcome. By recognizing and celebrating these differences the narrative fosters a sense of empowerment and pride in one's achievements.

Furthermore, the content explores how celebrating accomplishments contributes to cultivating a mindset. Seniors are encouraged to cultivate self-compassion and avoid comparing their progress, with others. By appreciating and celebrating their journey individuals can develop a relationship with exercise that extends beyond physical benefits.

In essence "Celebrating Achievements" becomes a narrative that inspires seniors to view their resistance band training journey as a series of victories of magnitude. It promotes an optimistic perspective, on accomplishments while fostering feelings of joy, motivation, and empowerment.

By incorporating the practice of celebrating accomplishments into their exercise routine older adults can establish a rewarding relationship, with resistance band training ensuring that the journey remains a source of happiness and well-being. The section on "Celebrating Accomplishments" in the book "Resistance Band Training for Seniors" tells a story that emphasizes the importance of acknowledging and rejoicing in the milestones achieved during the fitness journey.

At its core, this story encourages adults to develop a mindset that values not only major achievements but also the smaller victories encountered along the way. Focusing on reaching a distant fitness goal invites individuals to appreciate the ongoing journey and recognize each step forward as an accomplishment worthy of celebration.

Going beyond outcomes this content explores the benefits derived from resistance band training. It prompts adults to acknowledge improvements in well being increased energy levels, enhanced mood, and newfound confidence resulting from regular exercise. By broadening what is considered an achievement this narrative encourages seniors to cherish the impacts stemming from their commitment, to resistance band training.

The narrative also highlights how celebrating accomplishments can be a motivator. By taking time to acknowledge successes older adults create feedback loops that reinforce their dedication to fitness.

This positive reinforcement serves as a motivating factor that helps individuals develop an enjoyable exercise routine. Additionally, the content emphasizes the importance of embracing and celebrating the aspects of each person's fitness journey. It acknowledges that progress is personal and influenced by factors such, as starting points, goals, and obstacles. By appreciating and celebrating these differences individuals can feel empowered and proud of their accomplishments.

Moreover, the narrative highlights the significance of celebrating achievements in cultivating a mindset. It encourages seniors to practice self-compassion and avoid comparing their progress with others. By recognizing and honoring their journey individuals can develop a positive relationship with exercise that extends beyond physical benefits.

To summarize "Celebrating Achievements" promotes the idea that seniors should perceive their resistance band training journey as a series of triumphs regardless of size or scale. It fosters a perspective on achievements, which brings joy, motivation, and empowerment. By incorporating the practice of celebrating achievements into their fitness routine seniors can establish a fulfilling relationship, with resistance band training that enhances well-being.

Goal-Setting Beyond Physical Fitness

In the book "Resistance Band Training, for Seniors " the content takes a dive into the concept of goal setting moving beyond physical accomplishments. It encourages seniors to embrace an approach by considering goals that focus on their mental well-being, such as reducing stress and improving mood. By incorporating these objectives seniors can enhance their health and fitness in a more comprehensive and fulfilling way. The content explores the idea that goals encompass more than aspects of physical fitness. While strength, flexibility, and endurance are important in resistance band training it also prompts seniors to recognize and pursue goals that encompass emotional and social well-being.

Within this narrative, there is an exploration of goals well. Seniors are encouraged to set objectives related to function, memory improvement, and building resilience. This might involve incorporating exercises into their routine or engaging in activities that stimulate acuity. All these efforts contribute to a rounded approach, to well-being.

The importance of goals is emphasized in the context of resistance band training highlighting its impact, on mood, stress management, and emotional resilience. Seniors are encouraged to set goals that prioritize their well-being, such as fostering a mindset reducing stress levels, and cultivating inner balance.

Additionally, the content explores the aspect of goal setting for seniors. They are prompted to consider objectives that enhance connections, community engagement, and overall social well-being. This could involve participating in group resistance band workouts or incorporating interactions during exercise sessions. Setting goals that contribute to maintaining a connected life is also encouraged.

Furthermore, the narrative recognizes the significance of setting goals related to lifestyle improvement. Seniors are urged to consider objectives that align with their preferences and values. This can include achieving a work-life balance adopting eating habits or ensuring adequate rest and recovery. Ultimately "Goal Setting Beyond Physical Fitness" encourages seniors to view their resistance band training journey as an endeavor. By expanding the scope of goals to encompass emotional, social, and lifestyle dimensions individuals can create a framework, for overall well-being.

The section, on "Going Beyond Physical Fitness in Goal Setting" within the book "Resistance Band Training for Seniors" presents a story that encourages a perspective towards setting goals surpassing measurements of physical fitness. This narrative urges seniors to identify and pursue an array of goals that encompass aspects of their well-being.

At the core of this narrative lies the understanding that goals should not be limited to indicators like physical strength or flexibility. While these factors are important the content prompts seniors to consider objectives that encompass emotional and social well-being.

When it comes to goals the narrative suggests seniors explore targets related to function improvement, memory enhancement, and mental resilience. This may involve incorporating exercises into their routine or engaging in activities that stimulate sharpness thus contributing to a more comprehensive approach, towards overall well-being.

The narrative also emphasizes goals by recognizing how resistance band training can impact mood regulation, stress management, and emotional resilience. Seniors are encouraged to set goals that prioritize their well-being, such as cultivating a mindset managing stress, and finding inner balance.

Furthermore, the content explores the importance of setting goals, for seniors. Seniors are encouraged to consider objectives that enhance their connections and engagement with the community and overall social well-being. This could involve participating in group workouts using resistance bands fostering interactions during exercise sessions or setting goals related to maintaining a connected social life.

The narrative also extends to lifestyle improvement goals by encouraging seniors to align their fitness journey with lifestyle objectives. This may include achieving a work-life balance adopting eating habits ensuring sufficient rest and recovery time and overall promoting a lifestyle that reflects individual preferences and values.

In essence "Goal Setting Beyond Physical Fitness" presents the resistance band training journey as an endeavor. By expanding the range of goals to include well-being, emotional fulfillment, strong social connections, and a healthy lifestyle approach tailored to needs and desires; individuals can create a comprehensive framework for overall well-being. This narrative fosters a connection, with the resistance band training journey by promoting a sense of satisfaction and overall health and happiness beyond physical fitness metrics.

The final part of the chapter titled "Setting Realistic Goals" in the book "Resistance Band Training, for Seniors" brings together all the experiences and lessons shared, providing insights and encouragement to seniors who are embarking on their journey of resistance band training.

As we conclude this chapter it is crucial to emphasize the importance of setting goals as a foundation for a sustainable fitness journey. Seniors are reminded that achieving well-being is a process rather than a quick race and their goals should align with their unique circumstances in a practical and balanced manner.

The narrative highlights the significance of tailoring goals according to abilities while acknowledging that progress takes time. Seniors are encouraged to appreciate each accomplishment along the way understanding that every little step forward contributes to improvements in health and fitness.

Moreover, the conclusion emphasizes how goals can evolve as seniors progress in their resistance band training. As strength levels change personal preferences shift or lifestyles adapt it becomes essential to adjust goals. This adaptability ensures that goals remain relevant and motivating throughout a changing fitness journey.

Seniors are urged to approach goal setting, with optimism perceiving it not as a checklist but as an empowering tool that can be adjusted based on individual needs. The narrative emphasizes the importance of having a conversation, with oneself promoting introspection and self-compassion. The final section of this chapter aims to boost senior's confidence by assuring them that their goals are within reach and that their efforts are making a difference in their well-being.

In essence, the conclusion to the chapter on "Setting Realistic Goals" acts as a farewell encouraging seniors to approach the future with optimism and a practical mindset. By establishing goals celebrating accomplishments and adapting to the changing nature of their fitness journey seniors gain the strength and determination needed to navigate resistance band training while maintaining resilience, happiness, and a long-term commitment, to their health and wellness.

Chapter 10: Conclusion

In concluding "Resistance Band Training for Seniors," we celebrate the collective journey toward enhanced well-being, vitality, and strength. This book has been a guide, not just through exercises and routines, but through a holistic approach to senior fitness. As we close these pages, let it be a reminder that the journey doesn't end here—it's a continuum of self-discovery, progress, and resilience. Seniors are encouraged to carry forward the wisdom gained, the realistic goals set, and the milestones achieved. The versatility of resistance band training offers a sustainable and adaptable path for long-term health. Embrace the joy of movement, the empowerment of physical strength, and the holistic benefits that extend beyond the physical. May this book serve as a companion in the ongoing pursuit of a fulfilling and active life, proving that age is no barrier to the pursuit of wellness. Here's to the vibrancy that comes with every stretch, the strength found in each resistance, and the enduring commitment to a life well-lived through the empowering journey of resistance band training.

Recap of Key Takeaways

As we look back, on our journey through "Resistance Band Training for Seniors " it's important to summarize the insights that have been integrated into this guide. Throughout the book, we have explored the benefits of resistance band training for seniors in a manner. This summary serves as a tapestry weaving together the elements that seniors can take with them as they continue their pursuit of well-being.

At its essence resistance band training for seniors goes beyond exercises; it represents an approach to health that takes into account physical, mental, emotional, and social dimensions. The book has emphasized the significance of understanding the advantages provided by resistance bands – their adaptability and ability to cater to fitness levels. We have delved into the principles of resistance band exercises acknowledging the importance of form, gradual progression, and personalized adjustments.

Throughout our exploration safety considerations have been consistently highlighted. Creating a workout space that fosters comfort and minimizes risks has been paramount. Seniors are encouraged to prioritize warm-up and cool-down techniques as components, in preventing injuries and maximizing the effectiveness of their resistance band workouts.

The book serves as a guide, for seniors in choosing the resistance bands providing clarity on the various options available in the market. It empowers them to make decisions based on their fitness goals and personal preferences. Additionally, the book emphasizes the importance of creating a comfortable workout space recognizing how the environment contributes to a positive exercise experience.

The book thoroughly explores the foundations of resistance band exercises highlighting elements such as grip, hand positions, body alignment, and posture. Seniors are encouraged to pay attention to these aspects as they greatly influence both the effectiveness and safety of their workouts.

In addition to exertion special attention is given to breathing techniques as a part of resistance band training. The book emphasizes breathing and its role in promoting relaxation focus and overall well-being during exercise sessions.

A wide range of resistance band exercises specifically designed for seniors is thoroughly explored throughout the book. These exercises are thoughtfully tailored to meet senior's unique needs and strengths while maintaining simplicity without compromising effectiveness. Detailed explanations on form and execution are provided for upper body exercises like bicep curls and shoulder presses.

Furthermore, mindful breathing practices are introduced not only during exercises but also, as a practice that extends beyond them.

Older individuals are advised to incorporate breathing into their routines promoting a strong connection, between the mind and body which enhances the overall exercise experience.

The focus is on adapting exercises to prioritize health recognizing that personalization is crucial for maintaining a fitness journey. Seniors have been empowered to understand and listen to their bodies making adjustments that prioritize joint health and overall well-being.

A variety of standing upper body exercises using resistance bands have been provided as examples demonstrating the versatility of this form of training. From bicep curls to chest presses these exercises have been tailored to accommodate the needs and abilities of seniors offering a range of options that can be customized based on preferences.

The book emphasizes the benefits of health and flexibility training beyond just physical mobility. Seniors are encouraged to view flexibility as an interconnected aspect of their well being recognizing its role in promoting movement and preventing injuries.

The importance of weight-bearing exercises with resistance bands, in preventing osteoporosis and maintaining bone health is also addressed. Seniors are encouraged to incorporate these exercises into their routines as a means of promoting bone density and overall skeletal well-being.

The discussion has explored the realm of customized workouts, for health concerns among seniors highlighting the effectiveness of resistance band training in addressing needs. The book has provided insights into designing workouts that align with health goals covering areas such as joint health and cardiovascular fitness.

Understanding the aging process and how our joints adapt is crucial for effective resistance band training. Seniors are encouraged to approach their fitness journey with resilience adapting their approach as necessary.

The importance of knowledge for long-term wellness has been emphasized, acknowledging that staying informed is a tool in pursuing health. Seniors are encouraged to learn and adjust their resistance band training approach as they progress through stages of their fitness journey.

Additionally practical guidance, on incorporating resistance band exercises for health and flexibility has been provided. Seniors are guided through exercises that specifically target mobility offering a way to enhance overall flexibility and resilience.

Lastly, the narrative comes circle by emphasizing the celebration of achievements recognizing that progress takes forms.

Seniors are encouraged to not only celebrate their achievements but also the mental and emotional triumphs that come from their dedication to resistance band training. The approach emphasizes a view of setting goals urging seniors to consider not only physical fitness objectives but also ones related to mental sharpness emotional strength, social connections, and overall lifestyle enhancement. It is emphasized that goals should be adaptable and personalized to align with preferences and values.

In summary "Resistance Band Training, for Seniors" has served as a guide, mentor, and companion in the pursuit of an active life. Seniors are urged to carry forward the wisdom acquired the realistic goals set and the milestones attained. This journey is not an endpoint but an ongoing process of self-discovery, progress, and resilience. As seniors conclude this chapter of their lives they are poised to embrace the adventure with optimism, joy, and a steadfast commitment to their health and vitality through the practice of resistance band training.

The overarching narrative of "Resistance Band Training for Seniors" culminates in a call, to action; in striving for holistic well-being and vitality.

As we review the points it becomes clear that this guide goes beyond being an exercise manual. It serves as a resource, for seniors navigating the aspects of physical fitness, mental resilience, and emotional well-being.

Throughout the chapters, the guide emphasizes the versatile nature of resistance band training recognizing that fitness is not a one-size-fits-all approach. Seniors are encouraged to embrace progress with resistance bands understanding that every small step contributes to overall improved health.

The importance of safety is consistently highlighted, emphasizing the need to create a secure workout environment. This aligns to promote injury-free exercise experiences that support both physical and mental well-being.

Through resistance band training seniors learn about principles such as grip techniques, hand positions, body alignment, and posture. They are empowered to approach each exercise because the proper form is not a technicality but crucial for effective and safe workouts.

Furthermore, breathing techniques are presented as more than aspects of exercise; they are seen as gateways to mindfulness and holistic connections, between the body and mind.

Integrating breathing into your routine goes beyond the workout. It becomes a part of your life contributing to a sense of well-being. The book provides a collection of yet effective resistance band exercises that are suitable, for seniors. These exercises can be done while seated or standing tailored to meet their needs and strengths.

Exploring the integration of breathing reminds us that the benefits of resistance band training go beyond fitness. Seniors are encouraged to embrace a perspective on fitness acknowledging the interconnection between their mental and emotional well-being.

The importance of adapting exercises for health emphasizes the need for customization. Seniors are urged to prioritize their requirements and adjust their workouts accordingly. This adaptive mindset is demonstrated through examples of seated and standing body exercises highlighting the versatility of resistance band training.

The holistic advantages of health and flexibility training play a role in overall well-being. Seniors are prompted to view flexibility not as a goal but as a component of a comprehensive approach, to health that promotes functional movement and prevents injuries.

The focus now turns to preventing osteoporosis and promoting bones highlighting the importance of weight-bearing exercises using resistance bands. Seniors are guided on how to incorporate these exercises into their routines to improve bone density and overall skeletal health.

Tailored workout routines, for health concerns among seniors, emphasize the versatility of resistance band training. Seniors are empowered to design workouts that specifically cater to their needs giving them a sense of control over their fitness journey.

Understanding the aging process and the resilience of joints requires a nuanced approach acknowledging that an informed understanding of the aging body is crucial for effective resistance band training. Seniors are encouraged to approach their fitness journey with resilience adapting and adjusting as necessary.

The theme of education as empowerment emerges, advocating for learning and knowledge as tools for achieving good health. Seniors are encouraged to stay informed and adapt their resistance band training approach based on the stages they go through.

The incorporation of resistance band exercises for health and flexibility serves as an application of the principles discussed. Seniors receive guidance on exercises that specifically target mobility offering a targeted approach, towards improving overall flexibility and resilience.

The narrative comes into the circle as it emphasizes the celebration of achievements highlighting that progress can take forms. It encourages seniors to not only celebrate milestones but also acknowledge the mental and emotional victories that come from their dedication to resistance band training.

The holistic perspective, on setting goals resonates as a guiding principle urging seniors to consider not only their fitness objectives but also their mental, emotional, and social well-being. Goals are seen as benchmarks that can adapt to preferences, values, and the ever-changing nature of the fitness journey.

In summary "Resistance Band Training for Seniors" emerges as a guide that goes beyond fitness literature. Seniors are not simply encouraged to adopt resistance band training as an exercise routine. See it as a dynamic and empowering lifestyle choice. As they conclude this chapter seniors are ready to embark on an adventure with resilience, optimism, and a continued commitment, to their health and overall well-being. The empowering practice of resistance band training is not seen as a destination but rather an enduring journey of self-discovery, progress, and holistic wellness.

Encouragement for a Lifelong Commitment to Fitness

"Encouraging a Lifelong Dedication to Fitness" serves as a conclusion, to the story of "Resistance Band Training for Seniors " weaving together motivation, resilience, and the enduring pursuit of being. As we delve into this content we discover the encouragement that seniors require to foster a lasting commitment to fitness that extends well beyond an endeavor.

At the core of this chapter lies the understanding that fitness is not simply a destination but an ongoing journey—a journey that is unique to each individual, adaptable, and intimately connected to the ups and downs of life stages. The narrative begins by acknowledging that embarking on the path of resistance band training entails more than a commitment; it involves building an enduring relationship with one's health, vitality, and overall quality of life.

Seniors are urged to embrace the notion that age should not be seen as a limitation but as a perspective. They are reminded that their bodies, minds, and spirits possess the potential for growth and resilience. The content delves into the aspect of commitment by encouraging seniors to cultivate a mindset—a mindset that perceives every workout session no matter how modest, as a victory—an investment in their long-term well-being.

Furthermore throughout the narrative, an understanding of how commitment to fitness is dynamic, in nature—evolves alongside individuals changing circumstances and needs. The key point here is that commitment should not be seen as inflexible and rigid. Instead, it should be understood as an agreement that allows for adjustments, adaptations, and continuous growth, in one's fitness routine. Seniors are empowered to view commitment as an alliance that can be tailored to their needs, circumstances, and aspirations.

This content serves as a guide highlighting that the journey of resistance band training comes with its challenges. These challenges are essential for personal transformation. Seniors are encouraged to perceive setbacks not as obstacles but as detours on the path toward increased strength, resilience, and overall well-being.

It's important to note that "Encouragement for a Lifelong Commitment to Fitness" delves into the aspects of commitment. It invites seniors to recognize that commitment goes beyond exercises and extends to fortitude emotional resilience and social connections. This holistic approach emphasizes that committing to fitness means nurturing all interconnected aspects of well-being.

The narrative explores how community and support play roles in maintaining a commitment to fitness. Seniors are encouraged to seek companionship through group workouts, fitness classes, or by engaging with individuals who share their dedication, towards health.

This sense of community does not boost the responsibility we feel towards our fitness journey. Also adds to the happiness and satisfaction we derive from this shared experience.

By aligning our dedication, with well-being this content explores the long-term advantages of using resistance bands for training. Older adults are reminded that committing to fitness is an investment not only in their physical health but also in preserving cognitive function emotional well-being and an overall improved quality of life as they navigate through different stages of aging.

The narrative offers strategies for maintaining commitment over time. Older adults are encouraged to set adaptable goals that keep their exercise routine engaging and aligned with their changing needs. This may involve adding variety to workouts trying routines or seeking guidance to keep their commitment fresh and invigorating.

A significant aspect emphasized in the content is self-compassion. Older adults are urged to be kind to themselves recognizing that commitment does not require perfection. Instead, it invites an understanding of one's limitations and an appreciation for any progress made no matter how small.

Ultimately "Encouragement for a Lifelong Commitment, to Fitness" aims to empower individuals on their fitness journey. It conveys the idea that commitment is not something to be burdened by but a liberating choice and an investment, in one's current and future well-being. Seniors are encouraged to view resistance band training as a companion that adapts, evolves, and thrives alongside them throughout their years. The content serves as a testament to the enduring spirit of commitment—a lasting partnership with fitness that goes beyond age limitations overcomes challenges and propels seniors toward a future enriched by the benefits of dedication to resistance band training.

"Encouragement for a Lifelong Commitment to Fitness" unfolds as a tribute to the enduring essence of well-being resonating with the drive that motivates seniors towards dedicating their lives to resistance band training. At its core, this chapter serves as an uplifting beacon—a narrative infused with wisdom, resilience, and deep insights into the transformative power embedded within the fitness journey.

The narrative begins by acknowledging that embarking on the path of resistance band training is not a short-term endeavor but rather an important commitment toward long-term health and vitality. It recognizes that fitness holds significance beyond exercise routines for seniors—it represents a connection, between their body and mind.

This understanding forms the foundation for an exploration of the aspects that make up a lifelong dedication, to staying fit.

Age, which is often misunderstood as a barrier is presented from a perspective—a lens through which one can perceive their abilities and potential. The story encourages individuals to let go of limitations and embrace the idea that the body has an incredible capacity for growth and adaptation regardless of age. By doing this new viewpoint not only challenges societal stereotypes but also empowers seniors to approach their fitness journey with hope and possibility.

The psychological aspect of commitment takes the stage urging adults to cultivate a positive mindset. Each workout regardless of its scale or intensity is celebrated as an achievement—a step towards improved well-being. Older individuals are encouraged to view commitment not as an obligation but rather as a journey filled with victories reinforcing the idea that every effort contributes to long-term health.

Crucially the narrative explores the concept that commitment does not mean being inflexible. Instead, it emphasizes that commitment is an adaptable agreement that evolves alongside life stages. Older adults are encouraged to see commitment not as a contract but rather, as a partnership that accommodates changes, adjustments, and the natural ups and downs of life.

This perspective, on commitment, aligns with the process of aging emphasizing that the fitness journey is always changing and evolving.

Recognizing and acknowledging challenges is a part of this perspective. Seniors are reminded that setbacks should not be seen as failures but rather as parts of growth. The narrative reassures seniors that challenge opportunities to develop resilience and gain an understanding of their abilities. With this mindset, seniors are encouraged to face setbacks with resilience knowing that they are only obstacles on the path towards lasting well-being.

The concept of commitment is portrayed throughout urging seniors to understand that it goes beyond exercise alone. It also encompasses strength, emotional resilience, and social connections. This comprehensive approach presents commitment as a dimensional investment in overall well-being promoting a balanced and interconnected approach to health.

Community and support play roles in maintaining a commitment to fitness. Seniors are encouraged to seek companionship through group workouts, fitness classes, or engaging with individuals. The sense of community not only helps keep individuals accountable, in their fitness journeys but also adds joy and fulfillment through shared experiences. This supportive community becomes a source of motivation for seniors to persist in their commitment.

The benefits of resistance band training go beyond the gains. It emphasizes the long-term advantages of this commitment, for seniors. By engaging in resistance band training they can enhance their function emotional well-being and overall quality of life. This perspective reframes resistance band training as a practice that enriches aspects of life.

To maintain commitment over time practical strategies are suggested. Seniors are encouraged to set adaptable goals that keep their fitness routine interesting and aligned with their changing needs. The narrative also recommends incorporating variety into exercises trying routines or seeking guidance to bring freshness to their commitment and avoid monotony. These approaches help foster motivation.

Self-compassion plays a role in this process well. Seniors are encouraged to be kind to themselves and understand that commitment does not require perfection. Instead, it invites an understanding of one's limitations and an appreciation for any progress made regardless of its magnitude. This self-compassionate approach becomes a foundation for cultivating a nurturing relationship with one's fitness journey.

Overall "Encouragement for a Lifelong Commitment, to Fitness" goes beyond the narratives found in fitness literature. It presents itself as a dynamic and empowering conversation inviting adults to view resistance band training not as a task but as a lifelong companion—a valuable investment that adjusts, grows, and thrives alongside them in the colorful tapestry of their well-lived years. This story serves as a testament, to the enduring dedication—an enduring partnership with fitness that goes beyond age-related barriers, overcomes challenges, and propels adults toward a future enriched by the advantages of committing to resistance band training throughout their lives. It is a tribute to resilience an encouragement to embrace possibilities and a guide for adults as they navigate the journey of committing to fitness for life.

In the concluding pages of "Resistance Band Training for Seniors," we reach a moment—a moment that goes beyond the words on these pages and resonates as an empowering ending to a journey. This final chapter is more than a farewell; it is a call to take action a motivational climax that reverberates in the hearts of every older adult embarking on the empowering path of resistance band training.

As we bring this chapter to a close remember that the pursuit of fitness is an adventure—one defined by perseverance, adaptability, and an unwavering dedication to your well-being. The resistance band is not a tool, for exercising; it's like having a trusted companion on this journey. It adapts to your needs grows with your progress and stays by your side through every success and obstacle.

You've explored the basics of resistance band exercises mastering the nuances of grip, posture, and mindful breathing. You've also discovered how to modify exercises for health and embraced an approach that goes beyond just the physical aspects. Your dedication to fitness is not an obligation but a flexible commitment that aligns with the rhythm of your life.

Within these pages, you have witnessed firsthand the impact of resistance band training. It goes beyond benefits – it enhances mental clarity strengthens emotional resilience and fosters social connections. You've come to understand that age is not a limitation but merely a perspective and every step forward is cause for celebration – proof of an enduring spirit that defies stereotypes and embraces possibilities.

As you continue on your journey envision resistance band training as more, than a series of exercises; see it as a way of life – one that strengthens your body energizes your mind, and uplifts your vitality.

Investing in your life's richness engaging in a dialogue, with your health that evolves and flourishes with each passing day.

Your dedication to fitness tells a story of empowerment—a narrative that defies age limitations challenges notions and creates a path for a future defined by vitality and resilience. With every stretch of the resistance band, you're not merely exercising; you're scripting a chapter of strength composing a verse of endurance, and harmonizing well-being.

As you conclude this book carries the wisdom acquired the motivation. The commitment kindled. Your journey does not culminate here; it is a continuum—a tapestry awaiting to be woven with threads of dedication, adaptability, and the indomitable spirit that characterizes your pursuit of fitness.

Embrace each day, as an opportunity to nourish your body and stimulate your mind. Engage your spirit. Whether you are facing the sunrise of a fitness routine or basking in the sunset of an established practice always remember that every moment is a chance to celebrate the journey offered by resistance band training.

May your dedication, to staying fit be an inspiration, a tune that fills you with the happiness of being active the balance of good health, and the lasting energy that comes with living a fulfilling life. As you move forward in life let "Resistance Band Training for Seniors" serve as a guiding beacon—a wellspring of encouragement, insight, and a constant reminder that you can shape your fitness path both now and, in the years.

Extra Content

In the exploration of "Resistance Band Training, for Seniors " it's not about the exercises and routines; it's about understanding the tools that have become essential in this transformative fitness experience. Let's embark on a journey into the origins of resistance bands uncovering how these versatile and effective tools made their way into fitness.

Resistance bands, also known as exercise bands or resistance tubes can be traced back to the century. The birth of these powerful tools can be connected to the realm of rehabilitation and physical therapy. Initially created using tubing physiotherapists used resistance bands as a yet effective method to assist patients in their recovery.

The development of resistance bands gained momentum in the mid-20th century when their effectiveness was recognized not in rehabilitation but in strength training and general fitness. It was, during this time that these bands transitioned from being used in settings to becoming accessible tools for a wider audience.

The simplicity of resistance bands played a role in their adoption. Unlike gym equipment, these bands offered an affordable and space-efficient alternative.

Resistance bands have become incredibly popular in the fitness world not in rehabilitation centers but, in homes, gyms, and fitness studios worldwide.

A significant turning point in the use of resistance bands occurred during the 20th century when fitness professionals and trainers began to recognize their incredible versatility. These elastic bands, available in levels of resistance can be used for a range of exercises that target various muscle groups. They are particularly well suited for seniors as they provide a strength training method while being gentle on joints.

The usefulness of resistance bands extends beyond exercises. They are also highly valuable for improving flexibility promoting mobility and facilitating a range of motion – all essential factors for seniors who want to maintain or enhance their overall functional fitness.

Today resistance bands have firmly established themselves as a part of fitness routines, for individuals of all ages, including seniors. The market offers a selection of bands ranging from ones to looped ones with handles catering to different preferences and exercise styles.

As we incorporate resistance band training into senior's fitness journeys it's important to acknowledge the evolution these simple yet ingenious tools have undergone.

Resistance bands have come a long way starting from their beginnings, in rehabilitation to becoming versatile tools for strength and flexibility. Nowadays they have become allies for seniors who aim to lead more active lifestyles.

When seniors follow the exercises outlined in this guide they are not just embracing a fitness practice. Instead, they are participating in a time-honored tradition that combines rehabilitation, strength training, and the commitment to making fitness accessible to everyone. The simplicity of resistance bands is a testament to the idea that effective fitness tools can endure over time and continue to empower individuals on their journey toward well-being.

As resistance bands gained popularity, innovation, and technological advancements played roles in shaping their form. Manufacturers began experimenting with materials, designs, and features to enhance both functionality and comfort.

The traditional surgical tubing used in the days has evolved into a range of materials such as natural latex, rubber, and fabric. This diversification allows for variations, in elasticity, durability, and texture catering to the needs and preferences of users.

The introduction of handles has further expanded the repertoire of exercises that can be performed with resistance bands.

Handles were designed to provide a grip and enable movements to traditional weightlifting exercises. This innovative feature made resistance bands more versatile bridging the gap, between bodyweight workouts and conventional gym routines.

The introduction of looped bands, flat bands, and figure eight bands further expanded the possibilities of resistance band training. Each design offered benefits allowing users to target muscle groups and engage in a wider variety of exercises. Seniors in particular found these options advantageous as they could customize their workouts based on their fitness levels and goals.

The modern landscape of resistance bands also saw the implementation of color-coded resistance levels. This intuitive system simplifies the selection process by allowing users to quickly identify the level of resistance at a glance. Seniors can seamlessly progress through levels as they gain strength and confidence creating a fitness experience.

The convenience of resistance bands extends beyond their attributes. Online platforms and fitness apps have become resources for seniors offering guided workouts, instructional videos, and virtual communities that foster support and motivation. This integration with tools has transformed resistance band training into an accessible fitness solution.

In essence, the journey of resistance bands from their origins in rehabilitation to their form reflects the evolving nature of fitness itself.

These humble yet versatile tools have not stood the test of time. Also adapted to meet the changing needs and preferences of users ensuring their continued relevance, in the world of senior fitness.

As seniors begin their resistance band training journey described in this guide they are not only participating in a history of fitness innovation but also embracing a tool that has been refined and perfected over the years. The story of resistance bands is a testament to the enduring spirit of fitness—an evolving journey that spans generations making health and well-being accessible, to all including the community of seniors dedicated to a life full of vitality and strength.

9 798873 950003